HAIR GROW
SECRETS
LEARN HOW TO STOP HAIR LOSS & GROW YOUR HAIR
LONGER AND FASTER NATURALLY!
ENGY KHALIL

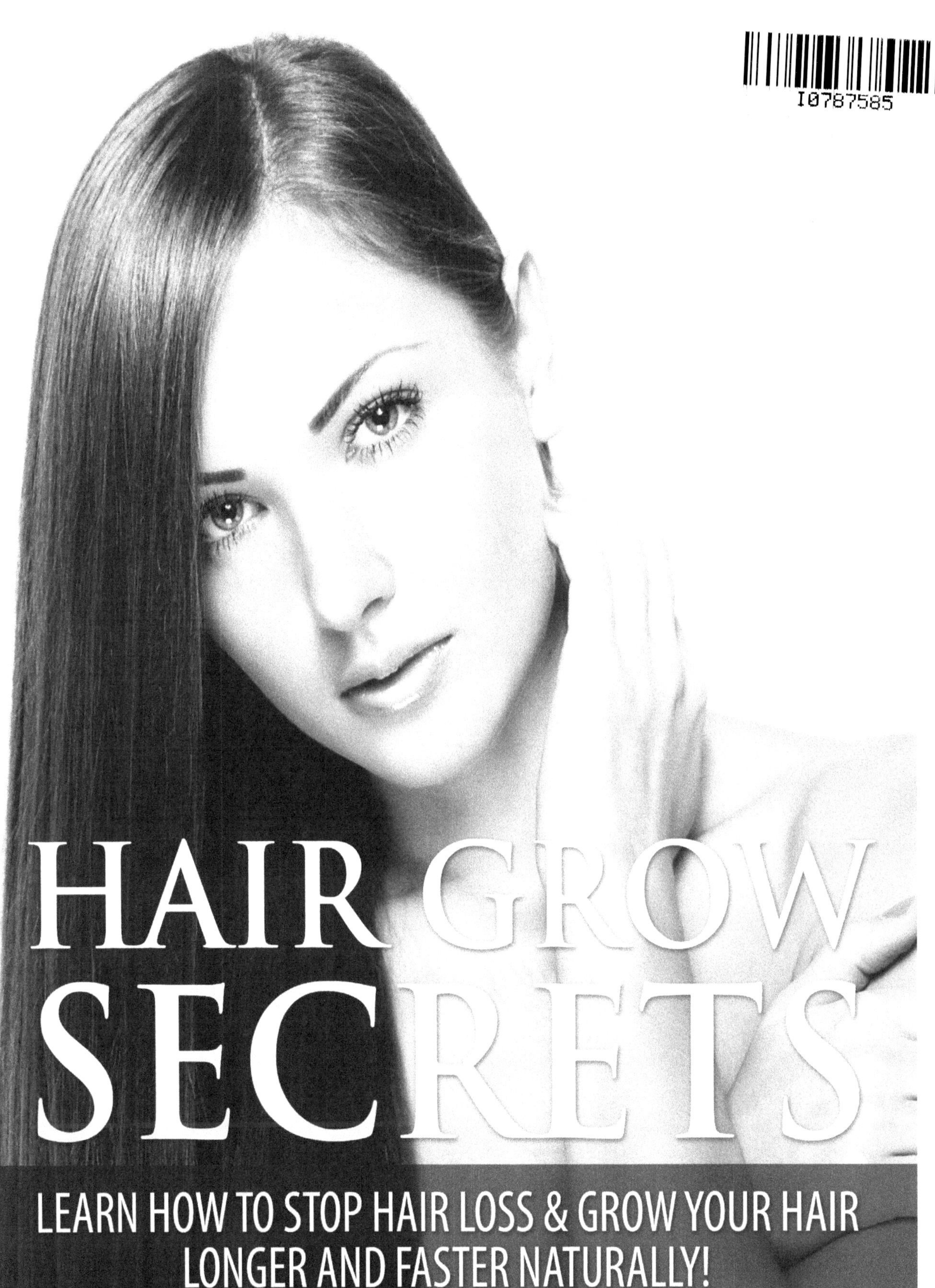

1

# Hair Grow Secrets

## How to Stop Hair Loss
## &
## Regrow Your Hair Faster Naturally!

by

Engy Khalil

Third Edition

# Table of Contents

# Disclaimer and Copyright Notification

The e-book Hair Grow Secrets: How to Stop Hair Loss & Regrow Your Hair Faster Naturally! is intended to provide helpful information and guidance to people who seek to improve their health. It discusses the numerous reasons and causes of hair loss in women and provides simple methods to combat the situation and grow their hair again. This e-book is intended for educational purposes only and addresses the health issues that cause hair loss. We do not provide guarantee for the efficacy or safety of any of the treatment options listed here. Readers are requested to consult their general physicians before approaching natural and artificial methods of treatment and remedies for hair loss.

# How to Use this Guide?

First i want to thank you for buying my program, everything you will read in this book comes from years of a hard work and many research as well as experience with thousands of my clients for these techniques. These techniques worked well for me and all my clients, they noticed changes in their hair as well as their whole health.

To get great results from this program, you should read carefully all the book from A to Z, don't skip any chapter or word as you will find ideas and solutions between the lines.

**Important Notes:** For the natural remedies please before trying any of these you must test a small patch to ensure you don't have any allergic to the ingredients.

Also if you have scalp scratches, scalp acne or inflammation in your scalp treat them first then try the Remedies.

If you are pregnant don't try any of these recipes and remedies until consulting your doctor.

If you have any allergies to some food that are in the natural recipes that means if you apply it to your scalp, you will get the same allergies in scalp, the solution is to replace it with another one.

# *What You Will Learn?*

As a busy working woman with many responsibilities, you may not have all the time in the world to tend to your tresses. Hair health and appearance is a common worry that plagues many women. Ranging from hair fall, dandruff, and dryness, weak and brittle hair can cause you a lot of unwanted stress.

If you have been exposed to the sun, pollutants and haven't had time to improve your lifestyle, now is your chance. This e-book has been designed to help you improve your overall approach to hair care and transform the way you care for your skin with the right foods entering your system, you can achieve strength and flexibility in your hair from within. The right nutrients can improve your tresses by providing resilience, shine and strength to deal with the everyday worries of work and home.

Apart from eating the right foods, exercising regularly can have a surprising effect on your hair.

By boosting blood circulation and ensuring a regular endorphin rush, you can bring down the stress levels in your body and allow your scalp to remain healthy.

With rich oxygenated blood filled with nutritional goodness reaching your hair roots every day, your hair care regimen is significantly shortened. No longer do you need expensive hair masks, conditioners and serums to keep them soft, shiny and strong.

Another way you can definitely improve your hair health is to align your needs to natural solutions. While off the rack hair products make tall promises, they only work from the outside. Filled with chemicals and undesirable toxins, these expensive products may make your hair look shiny from the outside but only damage the natural build of your tresses. This is why it is best to turn to natural remedies and therapies to nurture your hair. This e-book also highlights a number of natural ways through which you can strengthen your hair and make it shinier, longer and more resistant to the everyday wear and tear caused by pollution, dust, grime and UV rays.

# Introducing – Your Hair!

## How Does Your Hair Grow?

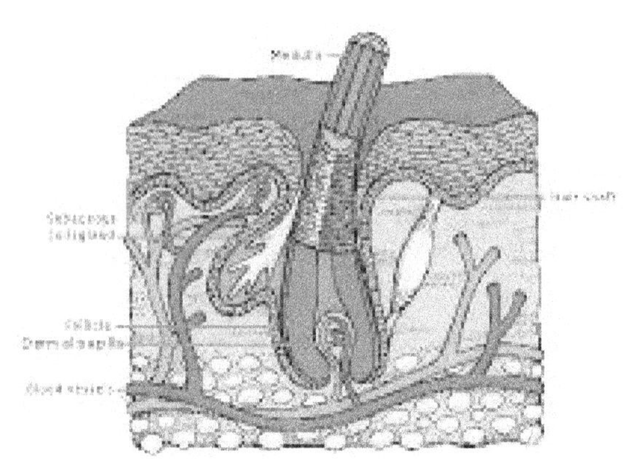

Apart from appearance and physical protection of the scalp, your hair has many purposes and benefits. Being more complex than imagined, hair is also essential in transmitting sensory information and to create gender distinction and identification.

Even in the fetal stage, hair follicles are useful. By the 22nd week, all hair follicles in the body are already formed. At this stage, about five million hair follicles are formed on the body.

About one million hair follicles are found in the head, with about 100,000 formed on your scalp. It is estimated to be the largest number of follicles an average human has. It is interesting to note that you do not generate or produce new hair follicles in your life. Another interesting thing you may have noticed about hair is that the general density of your scalp hair decreases as you grow into an adult. This need not indicate a reduction in the number of hair follicles, rather a spread out of the follicles since your scalp expands as your body grows.

# What is it Composed of?

The human hair is comprised of four distinct parts i.e. The follicle, Cortex, Cuticle and Medulla.

However, the follicle itself is made of many other parts. It is interesting to note that hair follicles are among the only two places in an adult human where stem cells are available.

On an average, your hair grows about six inches in a year and dies in the next four years. Your hair can also be divided into the follicle and shaft, the latter being visible over the scalp.

## Hair Follicle

The hair follicle can be defined as a tunnel like portion of the epidermal layer of the skin that extends all the way into the dermis. The structure of the hair follicle includes multiple layers with unique and separate functions. The base of your hair follicle is known as the papilla and contains blood capillaries that nourish your scalp and hair.

The living part in your hair strands, known as the bulb, is located at the bottom of the scalp and surrounds the papilla. The cells existing in the bulb divide every 1-3 days and are significantly faster than other cells in your body. It is this splitting of cells, which results in hair growth, and can vary from person to person.

The hair follicle is surrounded by inner sheath and outer sheath that protect and allow the hair shaft or strand to grow. The inner sheath ends below the oil glands, also known as the sebaceous gland or apocrine glands. The outer sheath on the other hand continues till the gland itself.

## Arrector Pili

A muscle named arrector pili is attached to a fibrous layer surrounding the bottom sheath at the lower part of the gland. When this muscle contracts; it results in the hair strands to stand up. Arrectores pilorum (plural) are generally made of minute muscle fibers. The contraction of these muscles is involuntary and is often induced by cold weather. That is why you often experience goosebumps in cold weather or even air conditioned environments.

# Sebaceous Glands

The same function commands the sebaceous glands to secrete oil and protect hair strands. The sebaceous gland is very important to maintain and protect hair health as it produces sebum, a substance that is known to condition your skin and hair.

When you reach puberty, your body starts producing more sebum and the production slowly reduces as your age. In fact, women are known to produce far less amounts of sebum in their body than men of the same age.

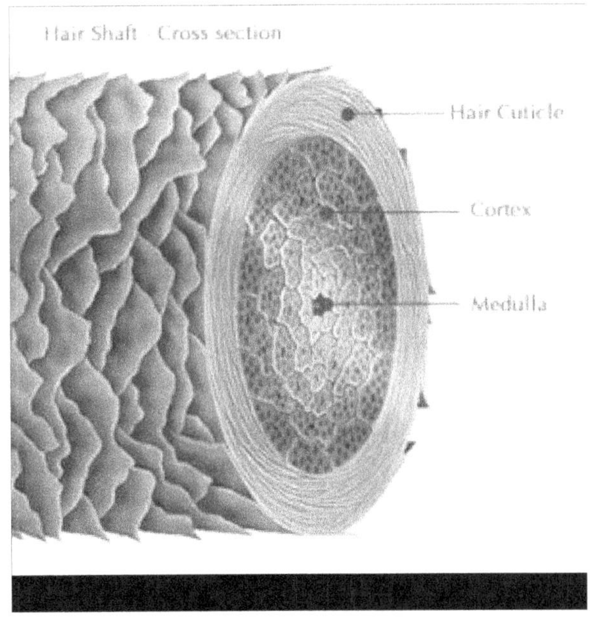

# Hair Shafts

Hair shafts are made of hard proteins known as keratin and can be divided into three distinct layers. The protein found in your hair is actually dead, making hair a non-living yet growing part of your body. The three parts of the hair shaft include the medulla, cortex and cuticle that are responsible for many distinctions in hair including color, strength, pigmentation, and so on.

**Medulla:** The medulla or medullary canal is located inside the cortex of the hair shaft and contains only air. Despite being an integral part of the hair shaft, medulla does not have any effect or influence on the properties or traits of human hair.

**Cortex:** The cortex surrounds the medullary canal and is situated inside the cuticle. Unlike medulla that does not have any correlation with the traits of human hair; the cortex is responsible for the weight, width and visual appearance of the hair.

It comprised of multiple braided fibers with pigments of red, yellow, brown and black.

The relative ratios of these pigments determine your hair color. This layer of the hair shaft is also responsible for many other traits of human hair including, thickness, straightness, and toughness, and is mainly made of water and protein.

**Cuticle:** While the cortex and medulla are found underneath the scalp, the cuticle is the protective layer found on the outside. The cuticle consists of keratin, a hard non-living protein and surrounds every strand of hair.

While the cortex is responsible for the waviness, straightness and strength of the hair, the cuticle determines the sheen. Well-maintained cuticles can reflect light effectively and give your hair a healthy and natural shine.

The cuticle is mainly made of scales that grow and point towards the tips and can include anywhere between five and 12 layers. It is mainly translucent and is not the main source of hair color. The cuticle protects the cortex layer inside and brings out the color based on its color pigment composition.

# The Phases of Hair Growth Cycle

Hair follicles function with repeated cycles of growth and each cycle can be broken down into three distinct phases – Anagen, Catagen and Telogen. Every single strand of hair on your scalp undergoes these three phases in each cycle and is completely independent of the other strands of hair on your scalp.

## Anagen Phase

This phase is also called the active phase or the growth phase of your hair. At least 85 percent of all the strands of hair on the scalp are in this stage at any given time.

The anagen phase is much longer than you might expect and runs anywhere between two and six years.
Hair roughly grows 10 centimeters every year on an average while the rate of growth can vary from person to person. In any case, the

total length of a single strand of hair is unlikely to grow after reaching the length of one meter. During this stage, the cells in the hair root are dividing at a rapid pace and new hair is formed quickly. The newly formed hair pushes the club hair up and out of the follicle.

In simple terms, club hair can be defined as specific strands of hair that have already passed the anagen phase. During this phase, your hair can grow about one centimeter every 28 days and remains active for several years.

Some people find it easier to grow their hair longer than others because of their lengthened active growth phase. The duration of the active phase of growth can decide how long your hair can be grown. The hair on your arms, legs, eyebrows and eyelashes have very short spurts of growth, lasting between 30 to 45 days. This is the reason why your body hair is never as long as your scalp.

## Catagen Phase

This phase is a transitional period between the growth and resting. Roughly three percent of your scalp hair is at this stage at a time, lasting between two and three weeks at a time. After the growth stops, the sheath in the outer root shrinks, attaching itself to the root of your hair. This process is known as the formation of the club hair. During this phase, the hair follicle shrinks to 1/6th of its normal length and lower part of the hair is destroyed. The catagen phase also sees the breakage of dermal papilla, resting below on the surface of the scalp.

## Telogen Phase

The Telogen phase is known as the resting phase. Roughly six to eight percent of all the hair on your scalp is at this stage at the same time. The Telogen phase lasts for about 100 days on the scalp. For body hair like eyelashes, eyebrows, arms and legs, the phase is much longer.

During the Telogen phase, hair follicles are at complete rest while the club hair is formed completely.

When you pull out a hair at this stage, you will notice a dry, hard and solid white material at its root. The Telogen phase also accounts for the normal hair fall. Roughly 25 to 100 strands of hair that are in this phase are shed every day and this is no reason for alarm.

During the Telogen phase, your hair stops growing, but remains attached to your hair follicle. The dermal papilla is also in place during the resting phase. When the Telogen phase approaches its end, a new anagen phase begins the next cycle.

The base of your hair follicle and dermal papilla rejoin and a new hair begins to form and grow. If the old hair in the same place has not already been shed, the new growing hair pushes it out, beginning the next growth cycle.

**Now that you have understood how your hair grows, we can move to understand exactly why your body has hair on your scalp and why hair loss is a serious problem to take better care of your health.**

# Main Functions of Human Hair

One of the primary functions of human hair is to protect your body and regulate temperature. With over five million hair follicles distributed throughout your body and scalp, your body works hard to maintain the right temperatures. While your body hair is mainly to control these temperatures, the hair on your scalp is to protect your skull.

Being one of the most important parts of your body, your scalp requires additional protection from the sun. It is also one of the few body parts that are exposed to maximum sunlight. This is why greater protection is required to ward off heat and radiations. With varying thicknesses, textures, lengths and properties.

**Human Hair Serves a Number of Purposes as Listed Below:**

1) Hair protects your scalp from external elements like sun damage and drying. It also protects your scalp from chapping from extreme wind and prevents dirt and dust from settling on your skin.

**For Example;** If you expose to the sun's rays in summer or use hair dryer (blow-dry) on thinning hair that is mean your scalp and follicles is very easy to damage and burn from the hot air. So hair is serving as a physical barrier between your skin and the external atmosphere and trapping warm air between the hair and skin. The insulation purposes of hair are useful in both cold and warm temperatures and ensure proper temperature regulation in your body.

2) The importance of hair for all women is that it can attract attention. Hair increase self-confidence of women and identify facial features. Sometimes the woman is not beautiful enough but she has a long lusters hair, she usually use her beautiful hair to serve as a compensation for ordinary face.

**Evident from the above, it's very important to maintain and protect your hair not only for the outer shape but also for healthy body and skin.**

# What Causes Hair Loss?

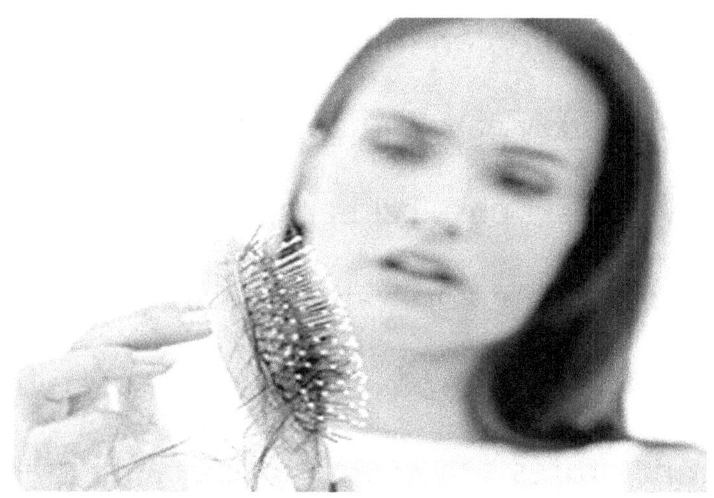

Hair loss is completely normal on a daily basis when you are showering, combing and styling your hair, it is completely normal to expect some amount of hair fall. Losing about 50–100 strands of hair per day is completely normal.

However, excessive hair loss can cause alarm as it more often a sign of an underlying problem and while it seems more frequent in men, it can also affect women.

If you are noticing significant hair fall and thinning, the underlying cause could be one of the following. In any case, it is best to pay a visit to your trusted dermatologist for help.

# There are Several Factors Which May Lead to Hair Loss and Thinning Hair:

- Stress

- Pollution

- Genetic hair loss

- Female pattern baldness

- Thyroid disease

- Lupus

- PCOS And Imbalance Hormone

- Improper diet

- Iron deficiency

- Impulse control disorder

- Alopecia Areata

- Aging

- Medication

- Excessive styling

- Scalp conditions

- Parasites

- Product Build-up

- Hair Tension

- Rapid weight-loss


In order to know what are exactly the causes of hair loss and thinning hair you need to look to your body health and scalp as healthy hair comes only from healthy body and scalp. It is important to read this chapter carefully that can help every woman to know problems and it may serve as a cautionary as to know what should to do and what should to avoid.

# Stress

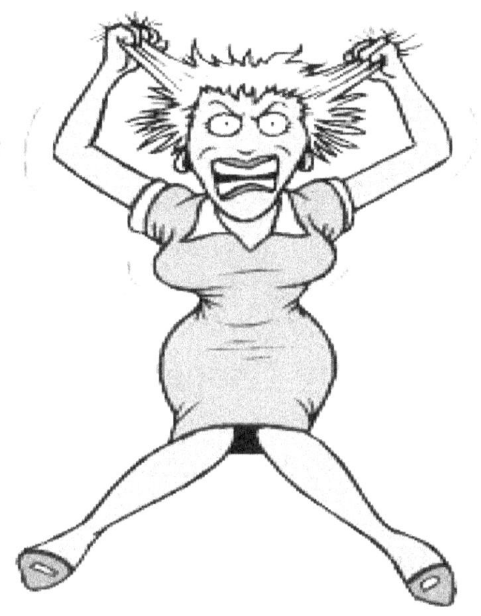

It comes as no surprise that stress can lead to hair fall. Everyday stress or extreme stress due to a one off event can trigger negative changes in your body, including hair loss.

Apart from regular stress, any event or experience that causes emotional or physical trauma can lead to hair loss. This can include anything from a severe illness, surgery, accident, leading to temporary hair loss. During a stressful event, your hair cycle undergoes a shock when most of your hair begins the shedding phase. In such cases, hair loss is apparently only after about 3–6 months. However, with the right diet and care for you mental and physical health, you can nurse your hair back to life as your body continues to recover and strengthen. The scientific term for this event is called Telogen effluvium, a phenomenon commonly observed after a major surgery, accident, illness, pregnancy or other events that cause extreme amounts of stress. During this phase, your hair shifts from its growing phase to the shedding phase much quicker than normal. While there are no tests to definitely identify Telogen effluvium, you can speak to your doctor about your hair loss systems and determine the functioning of the hair growth cycle.

# Tips:

- If the cause for Telogen effluvium is stress related, taking direct and indirect measures to reduce anxiety can benefit your hair.
- find unique ways to beat stress, whether it is taking up a new hobby, speaking to a therapist, working out or even meditating as this will directly influence the way your body recovers from stress. I tried these methods and got very good results.

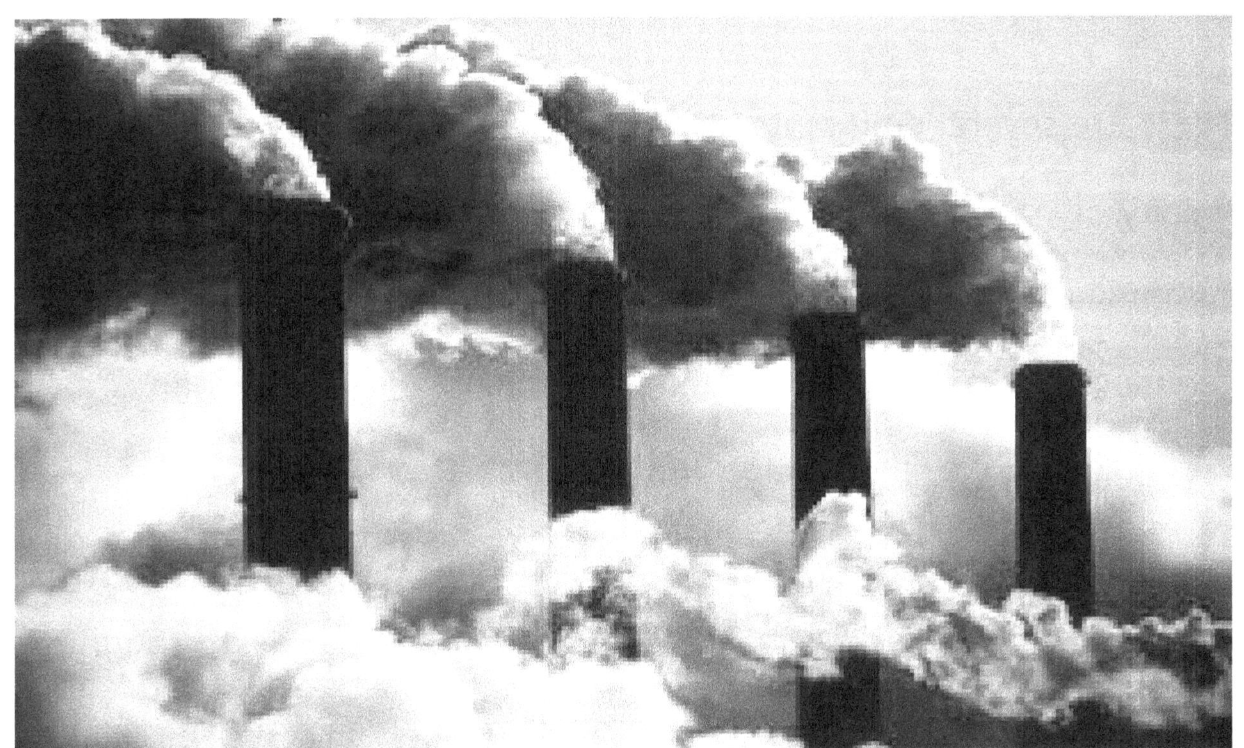

# Pollution

Pollution is a major reason behind the general depreciating health of women, even causing hair loss in some. Exposure to hot weather, smoke, and everyday pollution can have a drastic impact on your hair as chemicals and industrial pollutants affect its strength and integrity.

What makes it interesting is that even those who do not spend much time outdoors are at risk of pollution induced hair loss. If you work from home or indoors for long durations of the day, you may think yourself safer than others in terms of exposure to pollution. However, you will be wrong to assume so.

There are several pollutants in your home or office that can affect the quality of your hair. Anything ranging from cigarette smoke to common dust can influence hair loss. Cigarette smoke contains carcinogens that can easily damage your hair while the carbon content in regular smoke can damage your hair follicles.

Even if nobody in your vicinity is a smoker, you are at risk through common dust that contains microorganisms that lead to scaling and itching on your scalp. These changes are generally too minute to observe, but when left unchecked, can lead to serious problems.

In other rare cases, hair loss can be caused by pollution through food. Frequent consumption of preservative rich foods like junk food, packaged dinners and other processed items can introduce several undesirable chemicals into your body, causing a different type of pollution.

# <u>Tips:</u>

- In many cases, people have reported that switching to organic and more natural sources of food has significantly reduced hair fall. There is merit in avoiding fast food and other chemical filled products.


- If you are a smoker try to quit smoking, now you can find several solutions to quit smoking, when i was smoking i tried the <u>Artificial Cigarette</u> it helped me to stop smoking.


**Please Visit <u>http://fasterhair.net/artificial-cigarette</u> for More Details About Artificial Cigarette!**

# Genetic Hair Loss

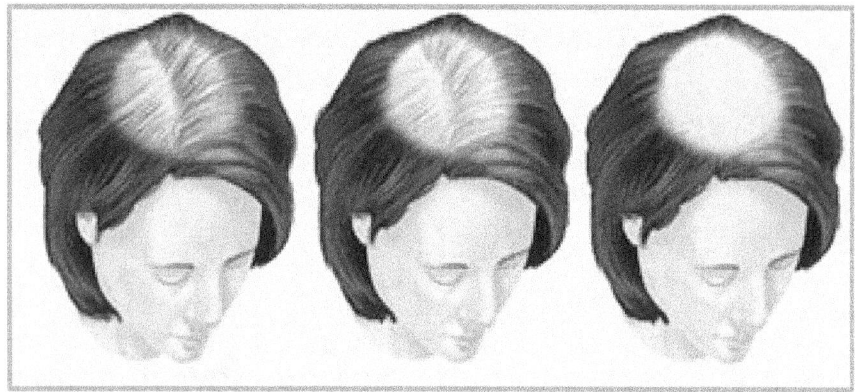

Genetic or hereditary hair loss is known as androgenetic alopecia and is one of the most common causes for female hair loss. The gene causing this form of hair fall can be inherited from either the mother or the father's family. However, if both parents have this form of hair loss, the chances of you facing genetic hair fall is much higher.

Some of the most common symptoms of hereditary hair loss include hair thinning behind bangs and crown. Even some young women in their 20s are known to develop this form of hair loss and they can become vulnerable to severe baldness if not treated immediately. Sometimes, the hair loss caused by genetics can diffuse and spread to the entire scalp.

# Tips:

You can slow down the hair loss with the right treatment as prescribed by your dermatologist. A common diagnosis method to determine genetic hair loss is to examine the pattern and test the hair follicles for signs of damage. Also, the natural hair remedies are very effective for these cases.

# Female Pattern Baldness

When defined in simple terms, baldness occurs when your hair falls out, but does not replace itself. While this phenomenon is very common amongst men, female pattern baldness is not well understood. It can be caused because of a number of reasons ranging from genetics, hormonal imbalances, aging, or menopause.

Symptoms of female pattern baldness are very different from male pattern baldness as the front hairline remains intact. However, hair loss and thinning most commonly occurs on the crown and top of the scalp and begins widening through the center.

Baldness in women rarely leads to complete balding as with men and only reaches as far as significant thinning and bald spots. Other symptoms of female pattern baldness are sores and itching on the scalp that are generally not obvious on sight.

☆ In most cases, female pattern baldness can be treated when checked on time and hair loss can be minimized.

# Thyroid Disease

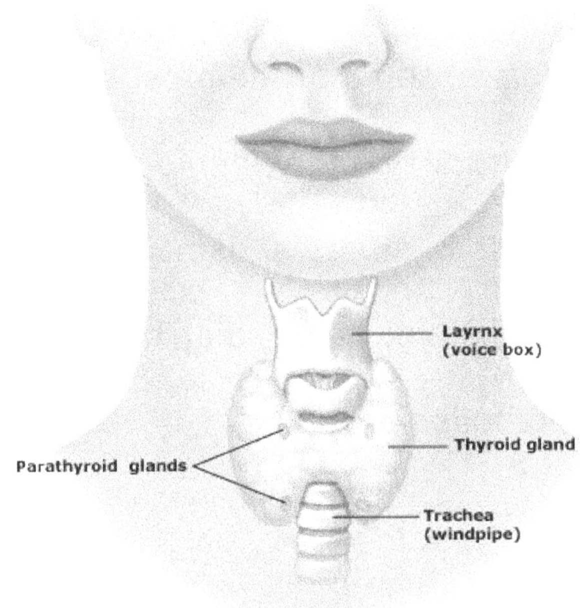



Thyroid disease or hypothyroidism affects millions of people all over the world; a significant number of them are women. The thyroid hormone is responsible for a number of functions including heart rate, metabolism and mood. It is also responsible for the way your body utilizes oxygen and energy to the growth and strength of your skin, nails and hair.

When your body does not produce enough thyroid hormones because of an under-active thyroid, it is known as hypothyroidism. On the other hand, if your body produces too much thyroid, you are said to have hyperthyroidism i.e. an overactive thyroid. Any imbalance in the production of thyroid can lead to hair loss.

In cases of hyperthyroidism, some of the most common symptoms include sudden weight loss, irritability, nervousness, heart palpitations, and weakness in muscles, damage skin, and sudden change in the appearance of your eyes, diarrhea, hair loss, and sudden increase in metabolism.

## Tips:

With the right medication to treat the underlying problem of hair loss like too much or too little of the thyroid hormone, you can reduce hair fall and improve its health and appearance.

# Lupus

A common chronic autoimmune disease, lupus affects millions of people around the world. The main problem caused by this disease is immune system begins attacking healthy tissues in your body. Lupus mainly strikes women in their childbearing years and can cause a plethora of side effects including hair loss, if not treated at the right time.

Some of the most telltale signs of lupus include headache, swollen or painful joints, oral ulcers and fatigue. In some cases, women are known to develop rashes across the nose bridge and tend to feel very sensitive when exposed to sunlight.

These rashes are often in the shape of a butterfly owing to its location. Other symptoms of lupus include swelling in the hands and feet, anemia, fever, chest pain and hair loss. Hair fall in particular can vary from person to person as lupus causes mild to extreme amounts of hair loss.

They can also accompany patching or rashes on the scalp. The condition lupus is often called the imitator as these symptoms are also found in many other health conditions, making lupus more difficult to diagnose and pinpoint.

## Tips:

Blood tests, tissue analysis and joint examinations are common tools used to determine lupus. If you are experiencing hair loss along with fatigue, joint pain and other related symptoms, it is wise to visit a rheumatologist immediately. Apart from oral medication, lupus can also be treated with topical creams and ointments.

# PCOS and Imbalance Hormone

Polycystic ovarian syndrome affects one out of four women around the world is a surprisingly common health condition. This condition is found in women and can start as early as the age of eleven. PCOS is normally caused by hormonal imbalances that lead to your ovaries producing an excess of male hormones and can often lead to infertility.

Some of the most common symptoms of polycystic ovarian syndrome include acne, facial hair growth, irregular periods, and ovarian cysts. Apart from an increase in facial hair growth, you may also notice excessive hair loss from your scalp.

## Tips:

PCOS can be diagnosed with a simple blood test for testosterone levels and sonar x-ray and can be controlled by Surgical or some medications that block or reduce the production of male hormones in women.

# Improper Diet

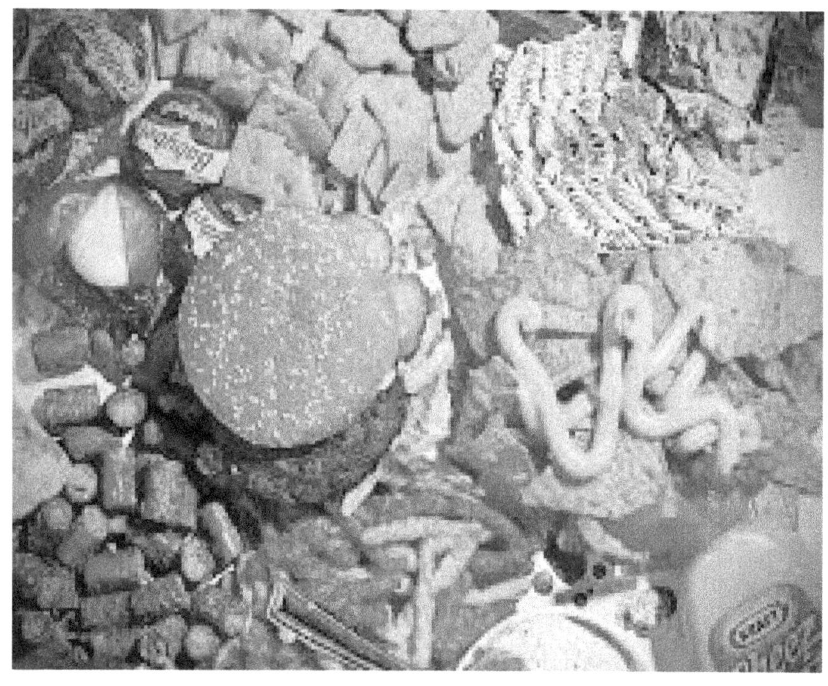

Vitamin supplements and medication can affect your hair growth. In fact, too much vitamin A can actually lead to hair fall. Fortunately, this process is easily reversible. Ensure that you stop consuming vitamin A supplements until it completely leaves your body and wait for your hair to grow back normally. Speak to your doctor on reducing your supplement intake and choosing natural food sources instead.

a Deficiency of vitamin B can also lead to hair loss. However like vitamin A, this problem is treatable and reversible.

Ensure that you find natural sources of vitamin B through non-citrus fruits, meat, fish and starch rich vegetables. You can also source healthy fats from nuts and avocados to improve the strength and texture of your hair.

Additionally, lack of protein in your diet can also lead to hair loss. If you don't source enough protein, your body starts rationing the available nutrition and shuts down hair growth. This change is visible only after a few months of the drop in, consumptions. Apart from health reasons, it is also important to consume adequate amounts of healthy protein through lean meats, low fat dairy products and fish.

# Iron Deficiency

Women who do not consume enough iron rich foods or experience heavy menstrual cycles are at a greater risk of iron deficiency. This condition occurs when your blood does not have enough red blood cells. As you may already know, red blood cells are essential to transport oxygen throughout your body and deliver it to organs, tissues and living cells. This oxygen gives you enough energy to function properly.

When you have iron deficiency, you could experience paleness in skin, fatigue, weakness, headaches, cold extremities, hair loss and loss of focus. Even the most minor of physical exertions could leave you tired and short of breath. Ask your doctor about taking <u>Iron supplement</u>.

**Please Visit <u>http://fasterhair.net/ironsupplements</u> for More Details About Iron Supplement!**

## <u>Tips:</u>

Hair fall caused by iron deficiency can be easily countered without treatment by simply improving your diet. Include iron rich foods like leafy greens, cereals, beef liver, fish, beef, and beans. When paired with foods in vitamin C, you can improve your body's capacity to absorb iron. Apart from natural foods, you can also opt for doctor-recommended iron supplements.

# Impulse Control Disorder

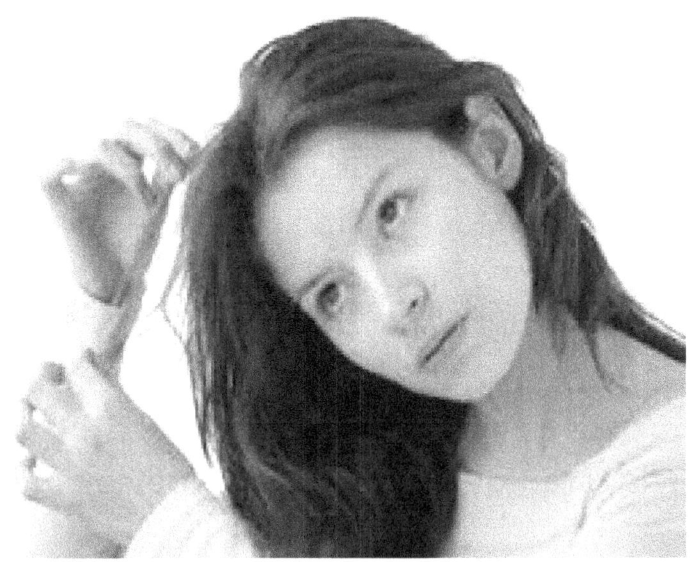

Impulse control disorder, also known as Trichotillomania, is a condition that causes people to pull their hair out. This disorder is similar to a compulsion and forces the person to constantly play with their hair or pull on them. Irrespective of the underlying causes of the condition, this constant pulling can strip your scalp of its protector. Trichotillomania is four times more common in women compared to men and can begin before the age of seventeen.

## Tips:

Behavioral modification therapy are the best way to control hair loss by eliminating the disorder from its root.

# Alopecia Areata

Alopecia Areata is one of the most common auto immune diseases where in your immune system attacks your hair follicles. Affecting millions of people worldwide, this disease occurs equally in both men and women. While the actual cause of the condition is depression or psychological trauma and sometimes the reasons are unknown, it is believed to be triggered by an existing or previous illness and/or stress.

Alopecia Areata can occur in three main forms. One of the most common symptoms of this form of hair loss is the appearance of smooth round bald patches on your legs, eyebrows or scalp. If you experience complete hair loss on your scalp, the condition is called alopecia totalis, while the loss of complete body hair is known as alopecia universalis. Tingling or irritation has also been noticed in affected areas.

Your doctor runs the diagnoses by observing the hair loss patterns and search for the percentage of iron in your blood. It is usually treated with a combination of medication and stress reducing measures.

# Aging

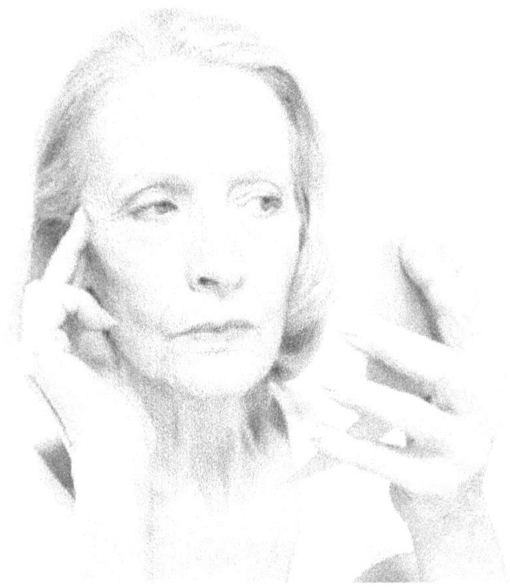

It is very common to notice hair loss after menopause for women over the age of 50. Most women don't know what is the reason of this hair fall in this age stage because the estrogen hormone level is decreased.

## Tips:

- If you are in your 45s or 60s and are experiencing hair loss due to aging, it is best to avoid any chemical hair products.
- Instead you can simply style your hair in a manner that conceals the patches and use Microfiber Keratin  it's excellent to cover thinning or bald area.

**Please Visit <http://fasterhair.net/microfiberkeratin> for More Details About Microfiber Keratin!**

- Also it is very important to follow a special anti aging diet. I strongly recommend to read The TOP 101 Foods that FIGHT Aging book by Mike Geary.


**Please Visit <http://fasterhair.net/mikegrearyantiaging> for More Details About this Book!**

# Medication

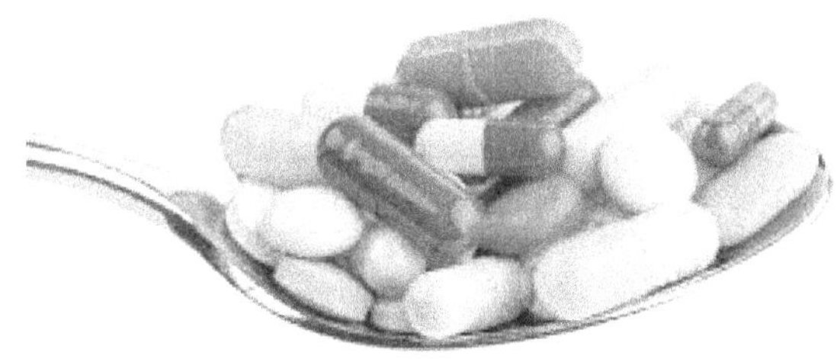

There are certain medications that cause hair loss. Some of the most common ones include high Blood Pressure drugs and blood thinners. Other drugs and medications that can lead to hair loss include anti depressants, gout, bipolar conditions medications it can cause thyroid problems which lead to hair loss, anti inflammatory drugs, as well as medicines for skin conditions like acne capsules and rheumatic problems. Anabolic steroids can also lead to hair thinning and is commonly consumed by bodybuilders and athletes. These steroids are known to have an impact on your body and can lead to the development of PCOS by increasing the production of testosterone and other male hormones in your body. Stop taking these medications as possible or at least ask your doctor to replace it with other treatment don't causes hair loss.

# Chemotherapy

Being a common form of treatment for cancer, chemotherapy can lead to excessive or even complete hair loss. It works on destroying cancer cells that are prone to divide quickly. Apart from destroying affected cells, the treatment also destroys other rapidly dividing cells found in your hair follicles. This is why most cancer patients experience a sudden loss of hair. In most cases, hair grows back after the treatment has been completely stopped. However, there are chances that the hair will turn out to be of a different color or texture. Owing to the noticeable hair loss, even your scalp skin becomes sensitive and irritated.

## Tips:

- One way of dealing with hair thinning and fallout during chemotherapy is to cut it very short or shave it completely. Despite being a drastic step, this has been proven to be easier for men and women to handle as they don't notice a sudden hair loss.

- If you are undergoing chemotherapy and are experiencing hair loss, there are a few steps you can follow to protect your hair from falling.

- It is ideal to switch to a gentle shampoo like organic or baby shampoo, these shampoos are free from harsh chemicals. Instead of using blow dryers or styling appliances, pat your hair dry or air dry it completely.

- Switch to a soft brush and avoid perming or coloring your hair. You can replace hair dyes by natural henna, it is chemical free and strengthening thinning hair.

- Use additional protection for your exposed scalp by wearing scarves or hats or human hair wigs.

# Excessive Styling

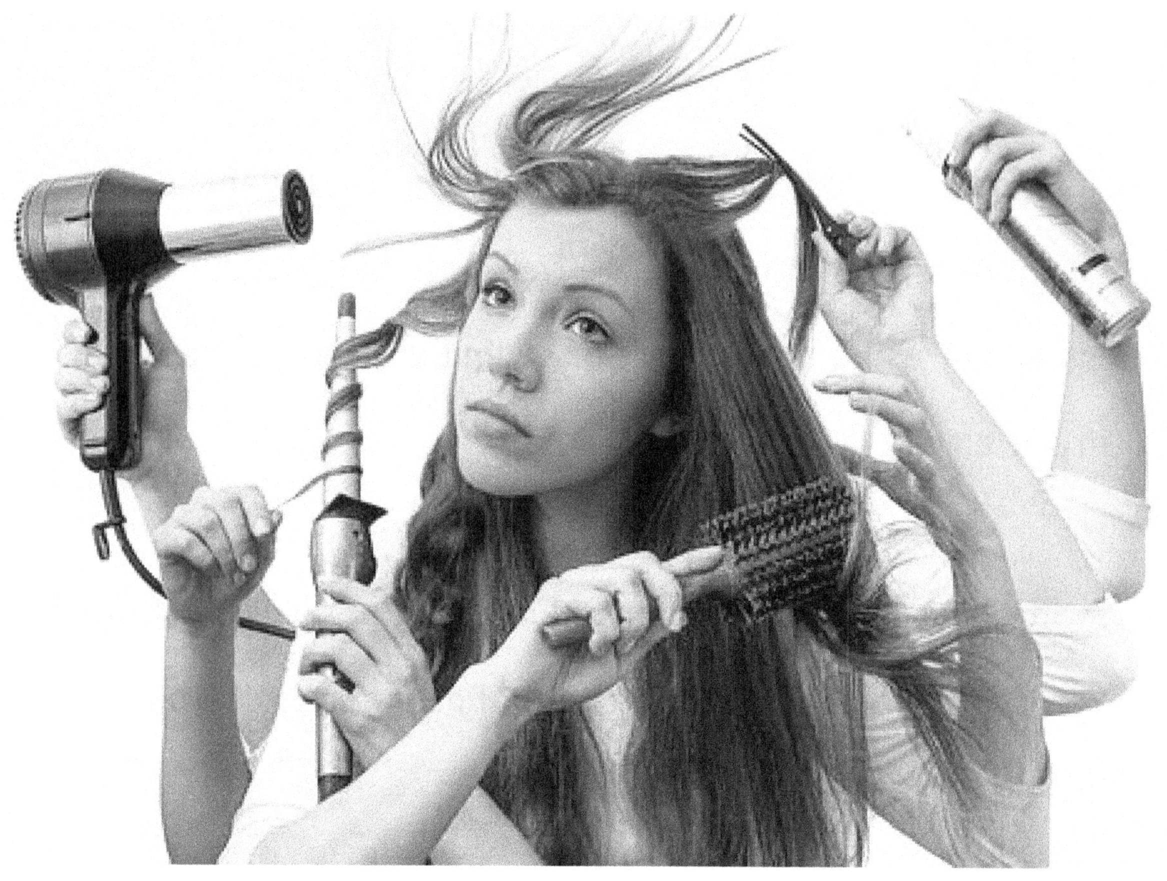

This is an unsurprising cause of hair fall. With the advent of chemical rich shampoos, hair dyes and other products, hair loss is an expected result. Owing to excessive dyeing, styling and shampooing, your hair will face a lot more damage than before, as these products harm hair follicles, hair cuticle, and also makes the scalp very sensitive. As well as the chemical content in the dye and shampoos paired with the heat emanating from hair dryers and straightening or curling machines, your hair becomes weaker and eventually falls out.

In most cases, the common cause for hair loss is the combination of keratin treatment, artificial coloring and regular blow drying. External damage caused by styling can lead to breakage and weakening of hair and compromise its strength, resilience and flexibility.

# Tips:

- To prevent damage caused by excessive styling, it is wise to stay away from appliances that cause overheating in your hair, whether you are straightening, curling or drying your hair.

- Set your hair dryer on cool or low settings and avoid using flat irons as much as possible.

- If you are insisting on using hair dyes, avoid choosing colors that are more than 1-2 shades from your original color.
  The more change in the hair dye, the more chemicals you need to complete the process. This exposure to heat and chemicals will definitely lead your hair to break easily.

- It is also a good idea to comb your hair immediately after you apply hair gel or spray as they are more prone to breakage after they set.

# Scalp Conditions

If your scalp is infected or otherwise unhealthy, it can become difficult to grow hair. Inflammation caused by scalp conditions can lead to an excess of hair loss and some of the most common problems associated with scalp skin include fungal infections like ringworm, psoriasis, and dandruff (seborrheic dermatitis).

The most common symptoms for these skin conditions include yellowish scales, greasy scalp, increased shedding. This could be the result of hormonal changes, excessive oil content in the skin or the yeast malassezia. Psoriasis is an auto immune disease that causes an excessive turnover of skin cells and produces white scales on your scalp. When pulled, they often bleed.

In cases of ringworm or other fungal infections, you could notice red patches on your scalp. Although these patches may diffuse over time, you could contract it through touching an infected animal or person.

# Tips:

- A thorough physical examination of your scalp can determine the type of skin condition that is causing the hair loss. In terms of infections, fungal and biopsies are most common.

- Medicated shampoos, anti-fungal natural recipes and/or creams and oral medications are commonly prescribed for ringworm and psoriasis.

# Parasites

Parasites can also cause hair loss and have devastating effects on hair, parasites are objects live inside the intestines and is involved in everything you eat. Parasites can pick up from pets like dogs and cats, eating uncooked food like meat and shellfish, eating pork, during Intimacy from person to another and Bug bites as parasites can introduce into bloodstream.

Symptoms are pallor, fatigue itching around the anus and colic especially after eaten. If you have these symptoms you should visit a doctor and do stool analysis. The treatments is available you can get rid of it very fast.

## Tips:

To avoid parasites infection you should wash your hands before taking your meal. Also it is very important to trim your nails regularly every week because the parasites live under nails, also brushing your nails with a clean brush everyday and cook meat and shellfish well.

# Product Build-Up

Dirt, sebum, sweat, most hair products and oils clog scalp pores which lead to hair loss, slow growing and hair breakage as well.

## Tips:

- You should to use a clarifying shampoo one time a month or at least one time every 45 days, this will eliminate and help get rid the hair of dirt, sebum, and debris from harsh chemicals and toxins that product build up.

- If you do not like to use clarifying shampoo apple cider vinegar rinse is the best alternative. Actually i love to use apple cider vinegar more than clarifying shampoo because clarifying shampoo makes my hair so dry.

# Hair Tension

Hair tension is pulling hair very tightly, it happens when you wear braids or buns or ponytails or wear clip or glue hair extension, too much hair tension causes thinning hair and bald area in the front of hair line and the crown area of the head which known as traction alopecia, it causes the induce follicular inflammatory, some women noticed a little bumps around the hair line and scalp pain.

## Tips:

- The best solution to grow these areas is to stop tightly and pull your hair back at all.

- The second thing is to massage this thinning area everyday before bed at least 5 minutes, if the pain and the bumps are still existing, it is important to pay a visit to the dermatologist for help.

- The third important thing is to try to use essential hair vitamins.

# Rapid Weight Loss

Rapid weight loss is no less than a physical trauma for your hair. Though weight loss may be good for you, dramatic weight loss most certainly is not. Apart from taxing your metabolism and burning out the lean muscles, rapid weight loss also damages your scalp and follicles.

Rapid weight-loss is triggered by crash dieting or starvation - your body is exhausted for energy and only focuses on vital functions like working your heart and brain. Result? You're thinner and so is your hair!

Further, hair is primarily made up of proteins. Lack of a balanced diet robs your body of its protein reserves and the body expends little or none of it on hair.

## Tips:

Aim for healthy weight loss, not more than two or three pounds a week. Ensure your daily consumption of protein doesn't fall below 46 grams. If your crash diet has in fact shocked your body, the hair loss will typically continue for six months , after which the body will resume normal function.

I know an excellent weight loss program called Fat Diminisher, you can check out here: http://fasterhair.net/fatd

# Understand What is Dandruff

Dandruff is a common problem that affects both men and women equally and lead to hair loss. When your scalp becomes excessively dry, you will notice dandruff flakes on your hair and shoulders.

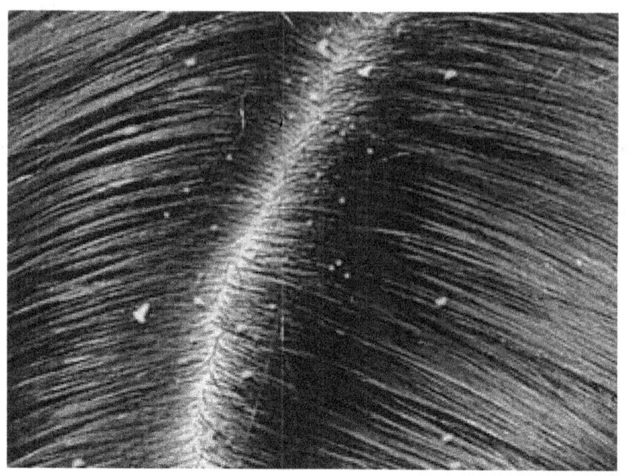

You can take many precautions to control and even eliminate this problem.

In the simplest terms, dandruff can be defined as the small powdery or flaky deposits that peel off from the skin on your scalp. Dandruff is usually associated with an unhealthy scalp, leaving it dry, sensitive and itchy.

In some women, dandruff is associated with unbalanced hormone levels while for many others, dry and cold winters affect the moisture levels in their skin. Regardless of the cause behind it, all cases of dandruff can be divided into two types – dry and oily dandruff.

**Dry dandruff:** It is usually associated with dry hair and scalp.

**While oily dandruff:** It is associated with oily skin. It's important to understand that both types of dandruff can lead to hair loss.

# What Causes Dandruff?

Before you attempt to solve your dandruff problems, it is important to understand the causes behind it. Like any other hair related issue to avoid the causes.

## Dandruff can be caused by a number of reasons including:

Poor health and diet, genetics, excessive scratching of the scalp, lack of vitamins especially B12, irritating chemicals, excessive combing or brushing, and infections.

# How to Treat Dandruff at Home?

There are several home remedies you can try to treat dandruff. Not only will successfully remove its symptoms, but you will also maintain a healthy scalp. Home based ingredients are gentle on hair and can improve the health and shines. However, the first step you should take when treating dandruff is to use an anti-dandruff shampoo, dandruff shampoos contains essential ingredients such as zinc and ketoconazole. Read the label to make sure it is for dandruff, be sure to choose a good brand. Also you can use a tea tree shampoo it can help.

**Please Visit http://fasterhair.net/anti-dandruffshampoo to Find the Best anti-dandruff Shampoos!**

# Natural Recipes
# to Get Rid of Dandruff

## Mixed Oils

✻ Try this natural recipe to get rid of dandruff, before you wash your hair on a weekly basis, apply a mix of organic olive oil and coconut oil to your scalp, then massage gently. This will not only remove dandruff, but will also nourish, moisturize your scalp and strengthen the hair roots, leading to less hair fall. You can get better results by heating the oils.

✻ Also **tea tree oil** is an anti-fungal substance, anti-bacteria, a natural dandruff treatment, unclogging hair follicles and an effective antiseptic. You can mix it with olive oil and/or coconut oil. Or you can add it to your shampoo.

# Tea Tree Shampoo

⭐ Add 10 drops of organic tea tree oil to 8 ounces of your regular shampoo, shake the shampoo bottle well before every use.

# White Vinegar Rinse

White vinegar rinse is the best solution for an itchy scalp and flaky dandruff, it 's my favorite rinse. Use this rinse before and after you shampoo your hair will make a great changes. Here is tips and instructions on how to use it:

## Before Shampooing:

Mix half a cup of white vinegar with a cup of water and massage your scalp with your fingertips. Avoid massaging with your nails to prevent further scratching your scalp and hurting your roots. Leave the mixture for up to 2 hours or more. For best results, apply this mixture overnight and let it settle into your scalp. In the morning, wash off the white vinegar rinse with lukewarm water and apply a gentle anti-dandruff shampoo.

## After Shampooing and Conditioning:

Add two tablespoons of white vinegar to about 500 ml of water and rinse your hair. Avoid rinsing with water after this stage. Dry your hair with a clean and dry towel by gently patting it. You can use a hair cream or leave-in conditioner if your hair is especially unmanageable.

**It is best to repeat this process about 2-3 times a week depending on the severity of the dandruff.**

# Tips for Fast Healing

* Wash your combs and hair brushes with white vinegar everyday to ensure that they are clean and eliminate infection.

* Change the towels and the pillows covers everyday with clean ones.

* Avoid scratching your scalp with your comb, or nails as that will only aggravate the problem.

★ Use soft brushes and wide combs to keep the damage to minimum.

★ Use your own hair tools, even at the hairdresser.

★ Avoid applying hair conditioners and/or hair masks directly to your scalp.

★ It is very important to avoid using 2 in 1 shampoos and cheap shampoos and conditioners.

★ If you still suffer of dandruff after 2 weeks using the anti-dandruff shampoo, mixed oils and white vinegar rinse, that's mean you have a stubborn dandruff and it is important to visit a dermatologist, the dermatologist will tell you about a medical treatments to solve this issue.

# Hair Management During Pregnancy

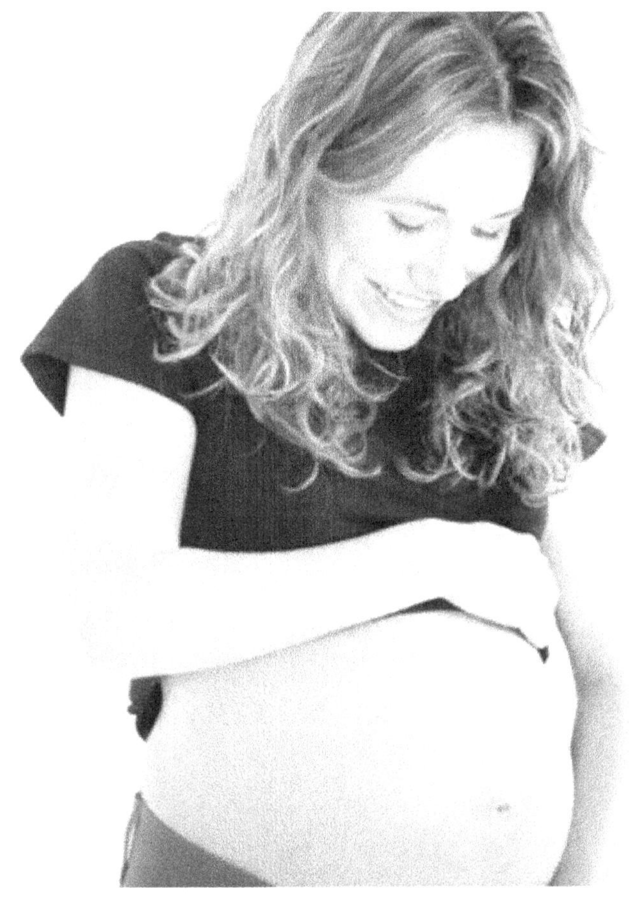

Managing your hair during pregnancy can be a tricky proposition as prescription medication is not always ideal. The following sections discuss numerous options that will help in taking care of your hair during pregnancy without having to turn to medication.

One of the most important steps you should take as a new mother is maintaining a healthy diet even after childbirth. It is important to understand that everything you eat has a direct influence on your hair and skin. Ensure that you eat as many raw fruits and vegetables as well as greens to get all the right vitamins and minerals. Turn to organic cosmetics like shampoos and conditioners instead of chemical ones as they are gentler on your hair. In many women, pregnancy has been known to change the texture of hair, making it more important to keep it moisturized and nourished.

Avoid using excess shampoo or blow drying your hair too frequently. Choose protein rich shampoos or herbal shampoos that naturally add volume to your hair and avoid the use of styling appliances that damage.

# Hair Loss After Giving Birth

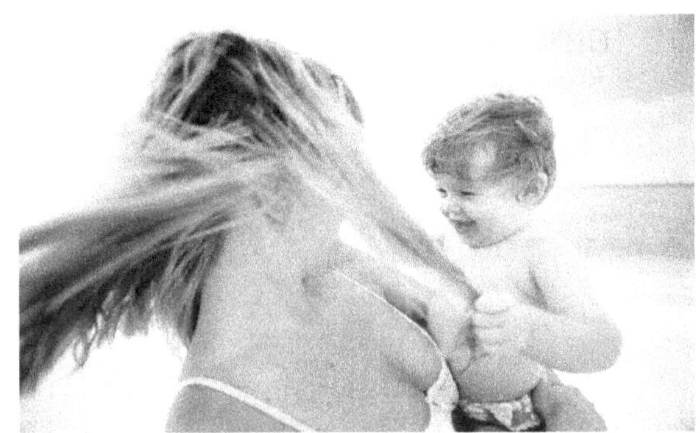

If you are still pregnant managing your tresses during pregnancy can be a tricky proposition as prescription medication or natural recipes is not always ideal. Because it may cause badly damaged a child's health. So please don't use anything even if it is natural before asking your doctor.

**If you are experiencing sudden hair loss after childbirth, do not worry as it is only temporary. Sudden hair loss usually occurs a few weeks after delivery and is not abnormal.**

## Why Does it Happen?

During pregnancy, your body is experiencing high levels of estrogen that tends to affect your hair growth cycle. By prolonging the growing phase, many pregnant women tend to experience thicker and lustrous hair. Since fewer hair are in the resting phase, the total hair fall during pregnancy is very low. After you have given birth, the estrogen levels in your body suddenly fall and a large number of hairs suddenly reach the resting stage. You may notice a lot more hair fall in the shower or when brushing. This unusually high amount of hair shedding usually normalizes itself in a few months as your body adjusts to normal hormonal levels.

It is also important to note that not all women experience this type of hair fall during or after the pregnancy. The intensity and length of hair loss varies with each woman and is more obvious in women with longer tresses. Hair loss is most apparent after a period of three months post partum as the hormones start returning to normal and your hair is allowed to fall. This sudden hair loss peaks between three to four months post delivery of your follicles take time to rejuvenate. Within the next six to eight months, you can expect your hair to return to normal.

## What Can You Do?

To be completely honest, there is nothing you can do to completely avoid hair fall. Being a normal and temporary phase for most women, there are other steps you can take to give your hair a healthier and fuller appearance. By maintaining the right diet, you can reduce hair fall. Speak to your doctor to ensure that your hormonal levels are balanced. This balance can help you maintain healthy hair. Eat foods rich in flavonoids and antioxidants that protect your hair follicles. Foods like proteins, fresh vegetables and fruits provide rich nutrition and promote hair growth.

# Scalp Massage

Scalp massage is gorgeous! It is the fastest and the easiest method to grow new hair and of course grow your hair longer faster.

## The Benefits of Massaging Your Scalp:

- Scalp massage boost better blood circulation to transfer nutrients, and oxygen and blood to the scalp and promotes new growth and strength follicles.

- It awaken and strengthen weak follicles. If your follicles are very weak but still alive scalp massage awaken it which makes it easy to produce new hair. Especially if you use an accelerator hair growth product or natural remedies.

- It speeds up your hair growth rate possibility and grow your hair longer faster.

- It assists in redistributing sebum oil to combat dry flaky scalps. So scalp massage is ideal for dry scalp.

- The scalp massage also helps you relieve stress and tension in the scalp and reduces headaches.

# How to Do a Scalp Massage?
## Scalp Massage Techniques

## The First Technique is Dry Massage:

First bending your head forward like the image below, then use your fingertips to make circular motions around your scalp. Start by rubbing your fingertips in clockwise, followed by anti–clockwise direction for 5 minutes. While the technique itself is not difficult, it is important to do a thorough massage of your scalp or at least thinning parts everyday to get the best results.

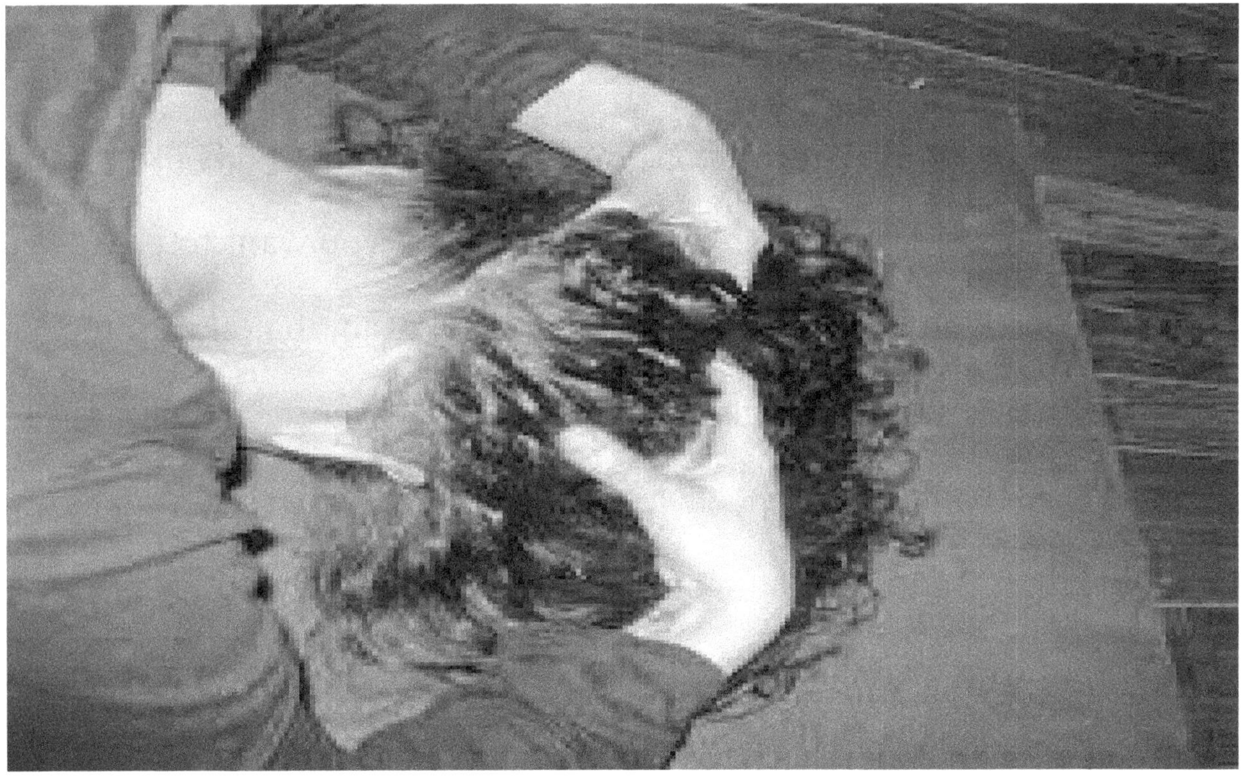

# The Second Technique is Oiling Massage:

Oil is a welcome part of a scalp massage as it helps lubricate and nourish the skin. The oils most ideal for a scalp massage include natural carriers like almond oil, coconut oil, jojoba oil, grape seed oil, avocado oil and olive oil. You can use any one or more of these oils, warm them and apply it gently through your scalp. These essential oils have healing properties that repair and nourish damaged hair. What's more, they also add a lasting fragrance that eases tension in your scalp and neck, while smelling divine.

The ideal scalp massage mix includes a handful of natural carrier oils like coconut oil or olive oil with a few drops of essential oils like lavender, peppermint, tea tree and eucalyptus. If you want to create a nuts and spices fragrance, mix one small bowl of jojoba oil with tea tree essential oils. You can also mix eucalyptus essential oil with olive oil for a fresh winter fragrance. Other popular scalp massage mixes include a mint fragrance that combines grape seed oil with peppermint essential oil. You can also go tropical by mixing lavender essential oil with coconut oil for a relaxing and soothing time.

# The Third Technique is Through Washing:

It is exactly like the second technique but you can do it when shampooing your hair.

# The Fourth Technique is Brushing Massage:

It is also very easy to do – Firstly comb your hair well to remove any tangles, then bending your head forward like the previous image and brush your hair with a soft brush; Starting from the back line of your neck to the front line of your bangs. You can also use an electronic massage brush.

* You can do this massage everyday at night with the first technique in morning.

The best time for a scalp massage is in the morning, just before bed. Choose a time of the day that is fairly relaxed and unoccupied so you can enjoy the relaxing effects of a thorough massage.

To get the best out of this practice, it is important to remain consistent. Choose a time and frequency that suits your schedule and stick to it – even if it is only for 5 minutes a day.

# Balayam

Apart from mainstream medicine and natural treatment methods, hair growth has answers in many alternative forms. a Popular and emerging method to deal with hair loss includes Balayam, an alternative form of reflexology that deals with hair growth.

This simple yet seemingly effective technique suggests that rubbing identical fingernails together with force can promote hair growth. Where there are several supporters and detractors for this technique, it is something that can be safely experimented with. Since the process does not involve ingesting any type of medication and can be performed in the comfort of your home, it is worth a try.

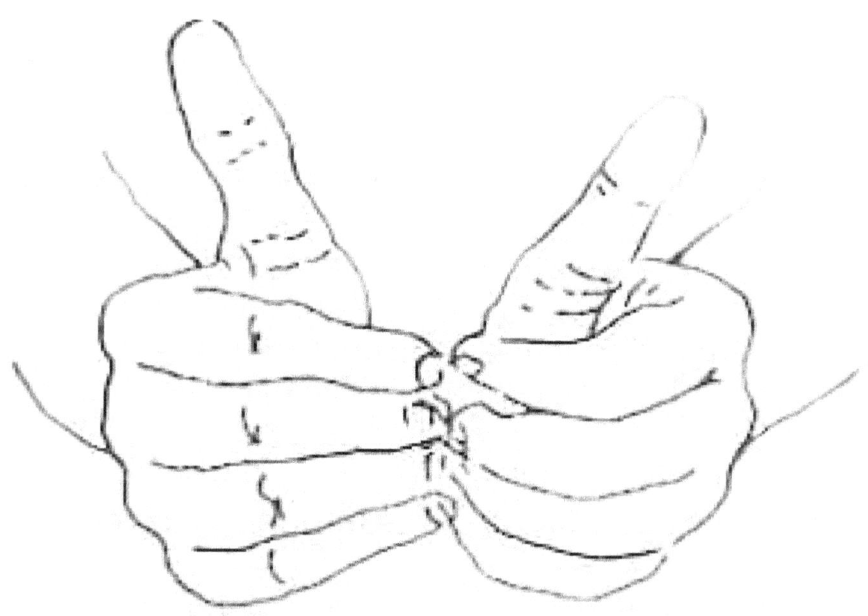

*Balayam Yoga Nails*

     72

# How Does this Procedure Works and How to Do?

This method suggests that rubbing your fingernails together for about 10-20 minutes every day boosts hair growth. It is important to avoid rubbing your thumbnails as it is believed to promote the growth of facial hair.

The method also suggests that the number of fingernails you rub is not a factor as long as you avoid rubbing your thumbs.
a popular claim by this method is that regularly practicing this technique can reduce bald spots and revive your original hairline.

The Balayam method is helpful in preventing hair loss and graying. Some also claim that practicing this method can restore the natural color of your hair.

It takes about 3-6 months to start showing signs of relief from hair loss and about one year to re-grow and replace the lost hair.

It considers some of the factors most commonly responsible for hair loss including medication,anemia, smoking, thyroid problems, hormonal imbalance, aging, genetics, protein deficiency, lack of nutrients, use of ammonium hair dyes and so on. Following the main principles of reflexology, Balayam believes that stimulating nerve endings located just under your fingernails can boost hair growth.

This happens when the nerves in your fingernails are stimulated, sending your brain a signal to revive unproductive or dead hair follicles. Rubbing your fingernails together can also boost blood circulation in your scalp and strengthen your hair.

The positive results of Balayam do not surface until a few months after you have begun the practice regularly. Despite the lack of scientific proof, Balayam is a popular practice to prevent hair loss. As it has zero side effects, those experimenting with this method will not face any health issues.

# is Balayam Method Effective for Everybody?

Balayam is not recommended for people suffering from high blood pressure as the practice can aggravate their condition. The same holds true for pregnant women who are advised against it as it could lead to uterine contractions as well as high blood pressure. Balayam is believed to lead to drowsiness and is not ideal to perform just before driving your car or during work hours. So, the best time to do the method is when you go to sleep.

If you recently have had appendicitis or an angiography, it is wise not to practice this method.

Balayam is also not advised if you have lesions, infected sores on your hands or suffer from diseased or brittle nails. Ensure that you do not rub the fingernails too vigorous as it can damage your nails permanently.

Apply a small amount of petroleum jelly, castor oil, olive oil or almond oil on your fingernails before you rub them together.

This will not only provide much needed lubrication and reduce friction, but will also moisturize your nails and make them stronger and healthier. Avoid rubbing your nails together for more than 20 minutes a day, splitting it into two 10 minutes sessions.

# Nutrition and Diet for Hair Growth

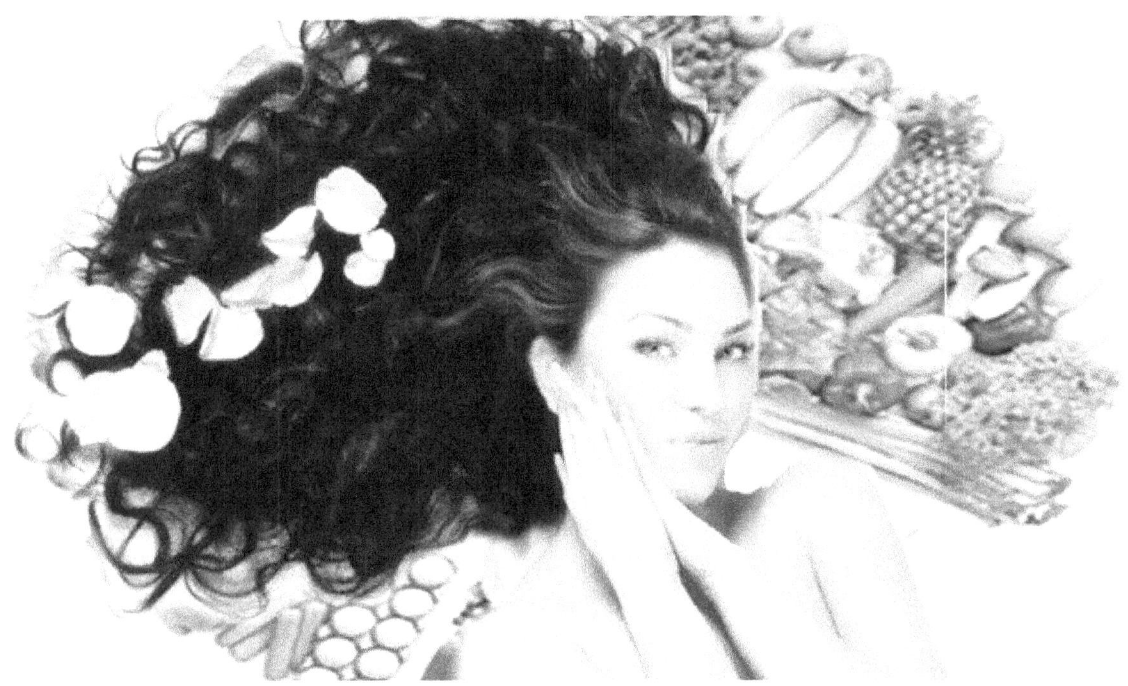

The current state of your hair is decided by several factors including your daily routine, stress levels, diet and exposure to pollutants. While you can use even the most expensive of hair products, they will not prove fruitful unless you maintain a healthy and well balanced diet.

Everything that you ingest is broken down by your digestive system and sent to different internal organs through the bloodstream. Watching what you eat is a beneficial practice whether you want to lose weight, become fitter or even enjoy healthier hair.

**Before you start learning the right diet for healthy hair, it is important to understand how your body handles nutrients. Your body prioritizes and distributes nutrients according to the importance of the organ.**

**For Example;** If your body is low on nutrients, it will economize and send these nutrients to essential body processes in your heart, brain, nervous system, digestive system and respiratory system. Your hair and nails are amongst dead cells that are the last to receive nutritional benefits of the food you consume. If your body does not have access to enough nutrients, your hair is the first to suffer since it is not essential for survival. Here are some nutrients that are essential to maintain healthy hair.

# Water

Your hair is 25 percent water, it would only make sense to drink enough fluids like juices and soup and plain water every day. If you are dehydrated and low on water, your hair may become dryer than usual. Water also transports vitamins and nutrients to the blood, which helps to get healthier hair. make sure that you drink at least eight glasses of water a day and carry a spare bottle wherever you go.

Also eat daily fruits and vegetables these foods are rich in water. You can focus on cucumber, lettuce, tomato, watermelon, peach, plum, kiwi and cherries.

# Green tea

Another effective drink is the green tea, it is rich of antioxidants, green tea can promote hair growth and reduce hair loss. Don't forget to supplement your hair regimen by drinking green tea as it removes free radicals, blocks dihydrotestosterone (DHT) which is the main reason for hair loss and purifies your bloodstream, which adds to the benefits of healthy hair.

# Protein

The main component of your hair is protein (keratin), human hair consists of about 80% proteins, making it an indispensable part of your diet. By ensuring that you consume enough protein every day, you can make your hair more healthy and strong. Low protein diets can often lead to slow hair growth, weak, dry and brittle hair, making hair loss inevitable. There are several great sources of protein you can find to complete your diet. Lean meats like fish, turkey, chicken, and eggs should be regularly incorporated in your meals. You can also supplement your protein intake with dairy products, nuts and legumes.

Adding protein supplements to your regime is a great way to nourish your hair, it is available in the form liquids, tablets, shakes. You can choose one of these as your choice.

# Iron

Low levels of iron in your body can not only make you anemic and weak, but also affect the quality of your hair. Baldness is a real danger if you are dangerously low on iron. Your hair roots and follicles are enriched with a rich supply of blood and when you face iron deficiency, you are at the risk of weakening your hair. You will also notice that your hair growth cycle is deeply disrupted if you do not source enough iron from your diet. Treat iron deficiency by choosing iron rich foods or taking iron supplements. Some of the best sources for iron in your daily diet include turkey, egg yolks, lean red meat, dried fruits, whole grains, spinach, and dried beans.

# Zinc

If you notice an increase in hair shedding, split ends and/or hair breakage, you may be short on zinc. This essential mineral is known to have an effect on the androgen levels in your body, a hormone that is often associated with hair shedding and hair loss. Some of the best sources for zinc include beans, lamb, beef, oysters, almonds, cashew nuts, walnuts, and pecans.

# Selenium

Another essential mineral necessary for healthy hair is selenium that protects your scalp from damage as it is an antioxidant. A lack of zinc and selenium can lead to a dry and flaky scalp and can easily be fixed with generous servings of shrimp, beef and eggs.

**Warning:** But eating too much foods contains selenium may cause toxicity at doses greater than 400 mcg/day and causes hair loss.

# Omega-3

Omega-3 fatty acids are essential for heart health and can have a profound effect on your hair too. These important fats are not synthesized by your body and are required to be [supplemented through pills](#) or natural sources. Healthy scalps are known to contain omega-3 fatty acids that are responsible in providing essential oils and keeping your hair hydrated. While you can get diet supplements for omega-3 fatty acids, you can also source these good fats from natural foods. Oily fish like sardines, herring, salmon, mackerel and trout are excellent sources of omega-3. If you are vegetarian, you can get your omega-3 through pumpkin seeds, walnuts and avocados.

# Lignans

Lignans, a disease fighting compound found mainly in flaxseed is known to improve hair health. It is also expected to slow down hair loss and can greatly improve strength and resilience of your tired tresses. Flaxseeds are best consumed in whole. Have about one and half tablespoons of flaxseed a day by adding it to smoothies, salads, oatmeal and other foods.

# Biotin

Although biotin deficiencies are rare and uncommon, a lack of this nutrient can lead your hair to become brittle and weak. This simple vitamin can ward off many health problems and is boon to your skin and nails. Some of the best sources for biotin include nuts, eggs, Swiss chard, legumes, brown rice and lentils. This water soluble vitamin B is also found in yeast, egg yolk, liver, whole grains and soy flour. I highly recommend to take Biotin 5000 tablets like GNC or Biotin 5000 injection from La roche to grow full head.

**Please Visit** http://fasterhair.net/gncbiotin5000 **for More Details About GNC Biotin.**

# Vitamin C

Vitamin C helps your system absorb iron and other essential nutrients. A deficiency of vitamin C can lead to weak, dry and brittle hair, making it an essential nutrient for healthy hair. Ensure that you consume enough vitamin C in your diet by eating a wide variety of fruits and vegetables. While you can opt for vitamin C supplements, this nutrient is best consumed from green peppers, broccoli, strawberries, leafy greens and citrus fruits.

# Vitamin A

Vitamin A is an essential nutrient that helps your body produce sebum. This important oily substance is necessary to condition and hydrate your hair. This sebaceous gland is a natural conditioner for a healthy scalp and the lack of vitamin A can lead to itchiness and dryness. Choose foods with high contents of beta carotene like sweet potatoes, carrots and pumpkins.

# Vitamin E

The damage caused to your hair can be reversed with adequate amounts of vitamin E. a Boon for great skin and hair, vitamin E-rich foods can help you reverse the effects of UV exposure and heat and provide protection for your hair. Dried fruit and nuts are the best sources for vitamin E and should be included in your everyday diet.

# Sulfur

If you want long thick hair, eat organic sulfur. By adding a small amount of sulfur to your diet, you will see a difference. Sulfur plays an important role in collagen synthesis and is vital consistent of Keratin, a strong structural protein necessary for healthy nails, skin and hair. It is found in milk, eggs, garlic and onions.

# Vitamin B complex

Vitamin B complex is necessary for the proper metabolism of fat carbohydrate and protein. These vitamins are also essential for skin and hair. A good Vitamin B complex capsule should look like this:

- Vitamin B 1 50 mg

- Vitamin B 2 50 mg

- Vitamin B 3 (Nicotinamide) 50 mg

- Vitamin B 5 (Pantothenic acid) 50 mg

- Vitamin B 6 (Pyridoxine) 50 mg

- PABA 30 mg

- Choline 30 mg

- Inositol 30 mg

- Folic Acid 400 mcg (micrograms)

- Biotin 200 mcg

- Vitamin B 12 (Hydroxy-cobalamin) 50 mcg

# The Top Foods That

# Promote Faster Hair Growth

## Vegetables

- Spinach
- Watercress
- Tomato
- Cabbage
- Broccoli
- Onion
- Garlic
- lettuce
- Artichoke
- Eggplant
- Zucchini
- Cucumber
- Mushroom
- Sweet potato
- Green beans
- Green pepper
- Carrot

- Strawberries

- Beets

- Parsley

- Radishes

- Turnip

- Ginger

- Celery

- Green coriander


# Fruits

- Avocado

- Grapes and Grape Leaves

- Peach

- lemon

- Orange

- Kiwi

- Apple

- Banana

- Cherries

- Coconut

- Grapefruit

# Proteins, Seeds .... etc

- Eggs

- Beef liver

- Fish – especially fatty fish

- Shrimp

- low fat dairy include milk, cheese and yogurt

- brewer's yeast

- molasses

- Oatmeal

- All Nuts – especially Almond

- Legumes

- Flax seeds

- Bran and bran bread

- Brown rice

- Lean meat

- Poultry

- Soybeans

- Cinnamon

# Skip These Foods and Drinks

For fast results you should skip the food and drinks listed below from your diet as it causes hair loss and slow growing. Here are:

- Caffeine

- Salt and Pickle

- Sugar

- Full fat foods

- Fast or junk food

- Processed food

- Canned food

- Alcohol

# Eat and Drink More From these for Fuller, Longer & Stronger Hair

**This is really incredible drinks, all you need for better hair is two cups.**

# Drink #1

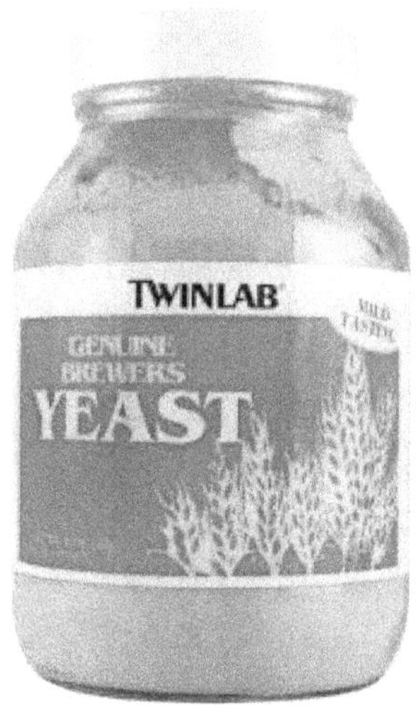

## Ingredients:

- 1 Tbsp brewer's yeast
- 1/4 cup of molasses

Mixing the brewer's yeast with the molasses and drink on an empty stomach. This drink is ideal for people who have anemia, have hair loss and want to grow long hair fast.

# Drink #2

Then after an hour drink this smoothie.

## Ingredients:

- 1 Banana
- 1 apple
- 3 strawberry
- 1 peach
- 1/2 cup of low fat yogurt or milk
- 2 handfuls Spinach leaves
- 1 Tbsp. Flax seeds
- 1 Tbsp. Oatmeal
- 2 scoops protein powder
- 1/2 cup of water (optional)
- 1/2 lemon
- 8 Almond
- 1 Tbsp. Honey or Stevia (optional)

Put all these ingredients into the blender, to become smooth, filtered or not, then drink. By drinking this juice everyday in the morning you will not believe how your hair grown and stopped falling completely as well as the energy you got.

# Raw Food
# The Perfect Salad

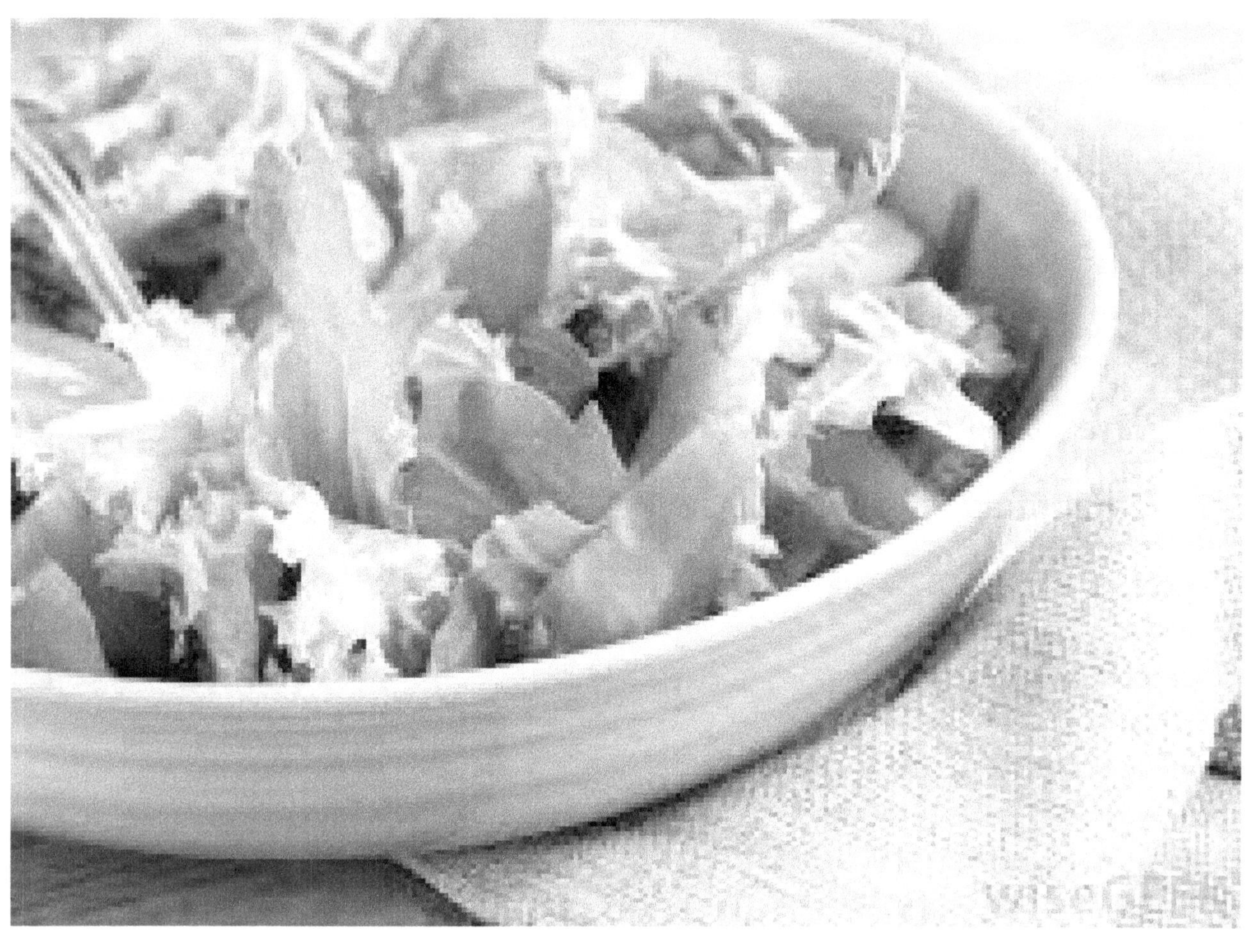

It's important to add this salad to your daily diet, this salad hydrates  your body, hair and scalp, as well as it speeds your hair growth rate. It is rich in vitamins, minerals, water and antioxidants. "Recommend to eat it daily".

# Ingredients:

- 1 Tomato

- Cabbage and/or lettuce

- Spinach

- One Beet

- 1 kiwi

- 10 Red Cherries

- 1 Minced clove of garlic and/or one red onion

- 2 Cucumber

- 2 Tbsp. lemon juice

- 1 Carrot

- 1 Green pepper or add all colored peppers

- 1 teaspoon of Grated Coconut (optional), recommend if you have

  dry hair and/or scalp and dry skin

- Some black pepper (optional)

- Some Cumin (optional)

- Some raw nuts

Cut all the ingredients to large or medium cubes, so as not to lose the vitamins, then add the lemon juice and stir the ingredients together. Eat this salad every day with lunch and proteins and you will see the big difference after few days.

# Faster Hair Growth Vitamins

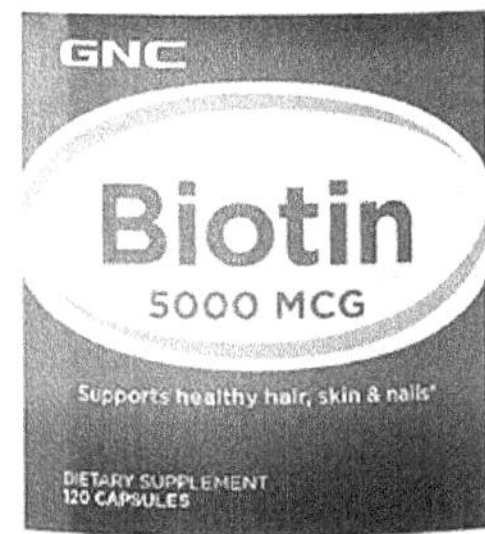

For fast results or if you have food absorbing problems you can take essential hair vitamins such as:

**Biotin 5000 and Bepanthen 5000 (Vitamin B5) muscle injections** with Pantogar capsules and vitamin C Fizzing drink or tablets. From 45 to 60 days you will see new hair growth starts to grow in the empty areas, guaranteed.

If these injections are not available in your country or you don't like injections, you can use Biotin 5000 ( highly recommend Biotin 5000 by GNC ), Vitamin B5 (Pantothenic Acid) tablets And Pantogar capsules.

- The complete treatment course is 4 months. Be sure to complete the course to get longer, healthier and thicker hair.

**Please Visit** http://fasterhair.net/gncbiotin5000 **and** http://fasterhair.net/Pantogarcapsules **for More Details!**

# Treatments and Remedies for Better Hair

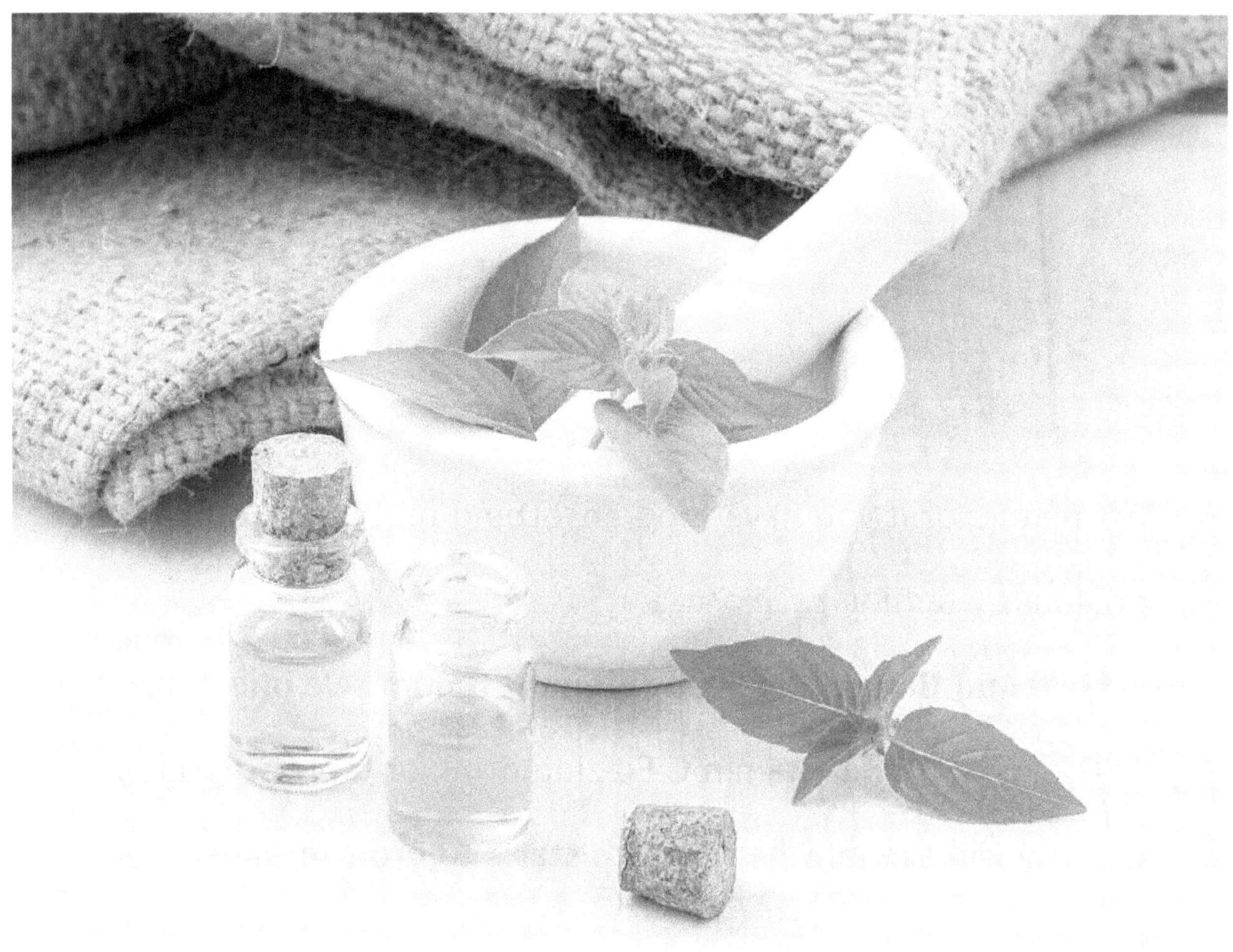

If you want better hair, there are many ingredients right in your kitchen that can restore the health of your damaged hair. Some of the most effective and affordable ways to rejuvenate your hair include natural ingredients that can be easily found and used. Here are some of the most natural options to nourish your hair back to health:

**Choose one or more from these remedies which suit your hair type:**

# Watercress the Magic Recipe

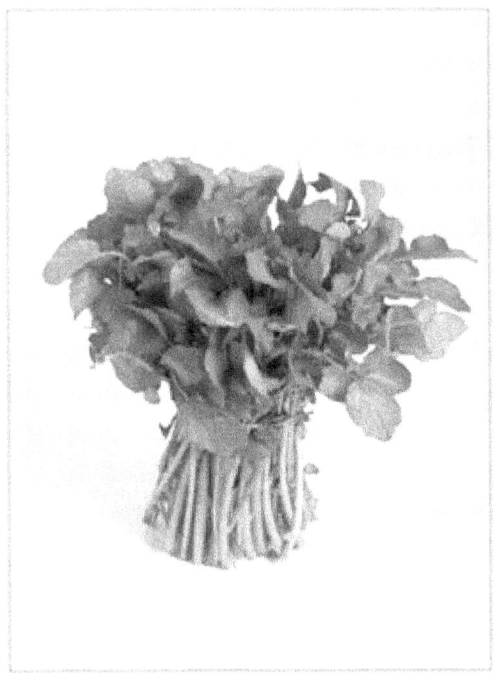

Watercress is rich in vitamins and minerals like Vitamins A, C, B-6, B-12, Potassium and Magnesium. **It is very effective to stop hair loss, grow new hair and grow hair longer.**

## Ingredients:

- 1 clean handful of full Watercress

- 2 or 3 cloves minced garlic

- 2 tablespoons pure castor oil

- 1 tablespoon olive oil

# The Recipe:

- Mix all the ingredients to become very smooth and creamy.
- Massage well but gently to a clean scalp.
- Cover your hair with a plastic cap.
- leave it at least 30 minutes.
- Wash with shampoo then apply the conditioner.

## Please Read these Lines Below Carefully:

- To stop hair loss and grow your hair more faster, do this recipe 2 to 3 times a week.

- To grow new hair in thinning parts, you must use it everyday, or at least day after day, for 60 days continuous without a break. After the first 28 days only you will see new hair growth started grow, as well as your hair will grow very long.

- Please Keep in mind that the results are according to your body's response and age.

**Also, it's very important to** supplement your hair regime by drinking everyday a cup of watercress juice **as it grows hair faster and longer and adds more strength to weak hair.**

## Here is the Watercress Juice Recipe:

Blend in the blender 2 to 3 clean handfuls of Watercress, 1/2 cup of low fat milk, some drops of lemon juice (optional), 1/2 cup of mineral or pure water (optional) and 1 teaspoon of honey. If you would like to add some fruits like; apple, cherries and Berries you can add. These fruits will nourish your hair, skin and whole body.

✳ **Drink this juice every day.** As for Vegetarians you can skip the milk.

# Onion and Garlic Juice Recipe

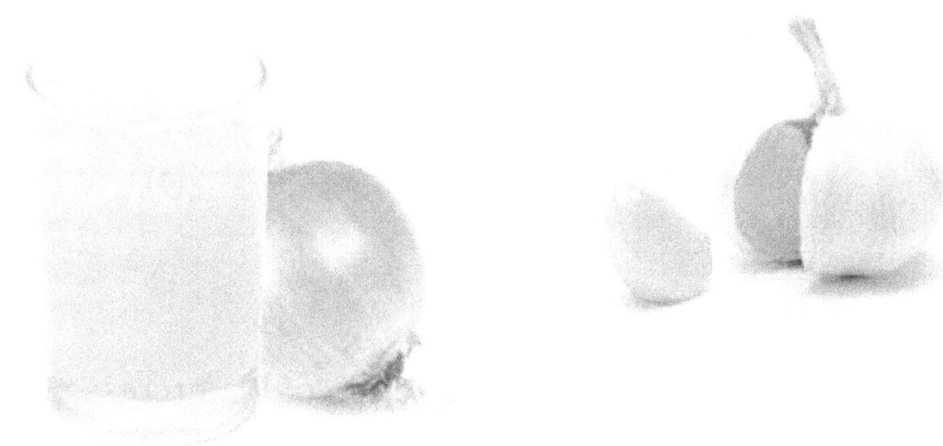

One of the oldest used method for fast hair growth and hair loss is the onion and garlic juice, both plants are rich in sulfur that improves hair growth and increase collagen levels in the body.

Widely known for a number of herbal benefits, garlic is a boon for hair growth. Apart from reducing the hair loss, garlic also boosts the regeneration and growth of new hair by promoting scalp circulation.

Here are amazing recipes should try:

 

# The Recipe:

- You can use 2 to 4 cloves of minced garlic and one red onion, chop them into small pieces, blend into the blender and squeeze out the juice.

- Apply this juice to your scalp only, massage gently, cover with a plastic cap and allow it to rest for about 2 hours.

- Rinse off the juice with a mild shampoo and warm water. Then conditioning.

## Here is Another Effective Garlic Remedy:

# The Recipe:

Boil a few crushed garlic cloves in coconut oil or olive oil and apply it on your roots. Apply this mixture three times a week for lasting benefits.

**Note:** I tried an expensive garlic hair lotion and i have found that the results was better by using natural garlic recipes and more effective than garlic treatment lotion.

# Nettle Tonic

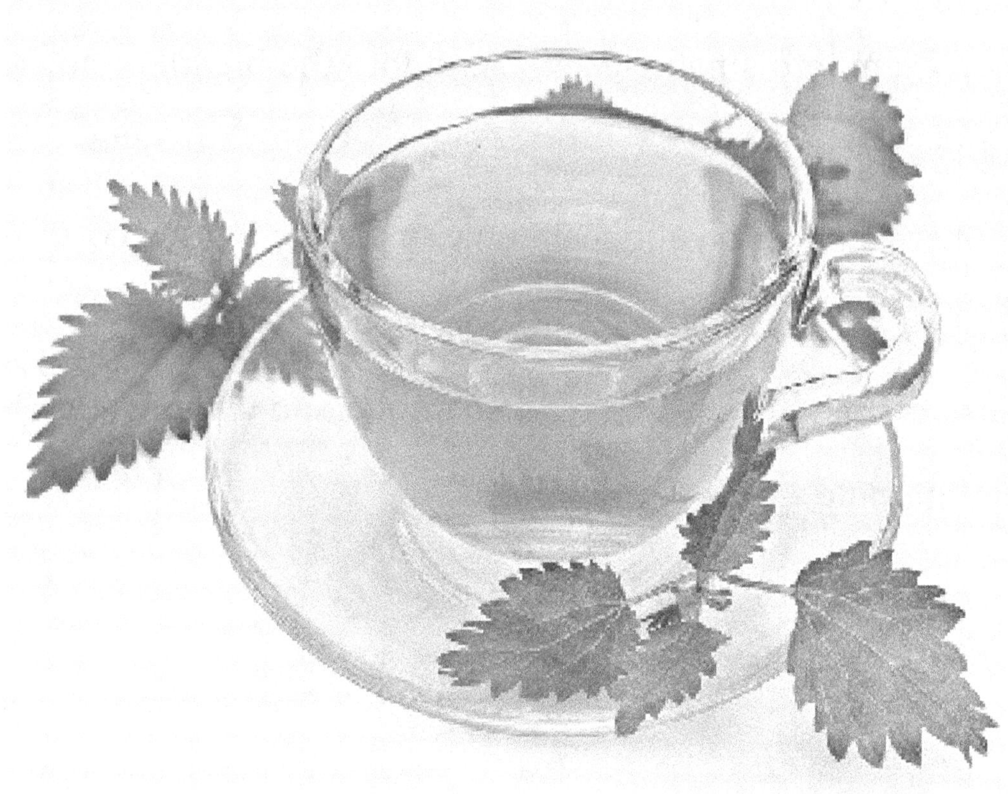

Nettle herbal is rich in vitamins and minerals like A, C, K, potassium, calcium, magnesium, protein, iron and chlorophyll.

It improves blood circulation, encourages hair growth, prevents shedding and thickens hair. It is also considered the best natural treatment to combat imbalance hormone, it inhibits testosterone from being turned into DHT, which makes hair follicles don't produces new hair. Nettle is available in several hair growth products on the market, like shampoos and lotions, you can do this natural recipe at home instead of buying expensive Nettle products.

# The Recipe:

- Add 4 tablespoon of Nettle leaves and 4 tablespoon of white wine vinegar to a cup of water.

- Boil all the ingredients on low heat. After boiling add 2 drops of lavender oil and/or 2 drops of rosemary oil.

- Let the tonic to cool then shake the mixture well before using, then apply the tonic to clean hair, massage the mixture into your scalp gently, leave it overnight or at least 2 hours and wash in the second day.

- Use this tonic 2 to 3 times a week.

- For best results you can drink one cup of nettle tea everyday that can improve the results.

# Potato Juice

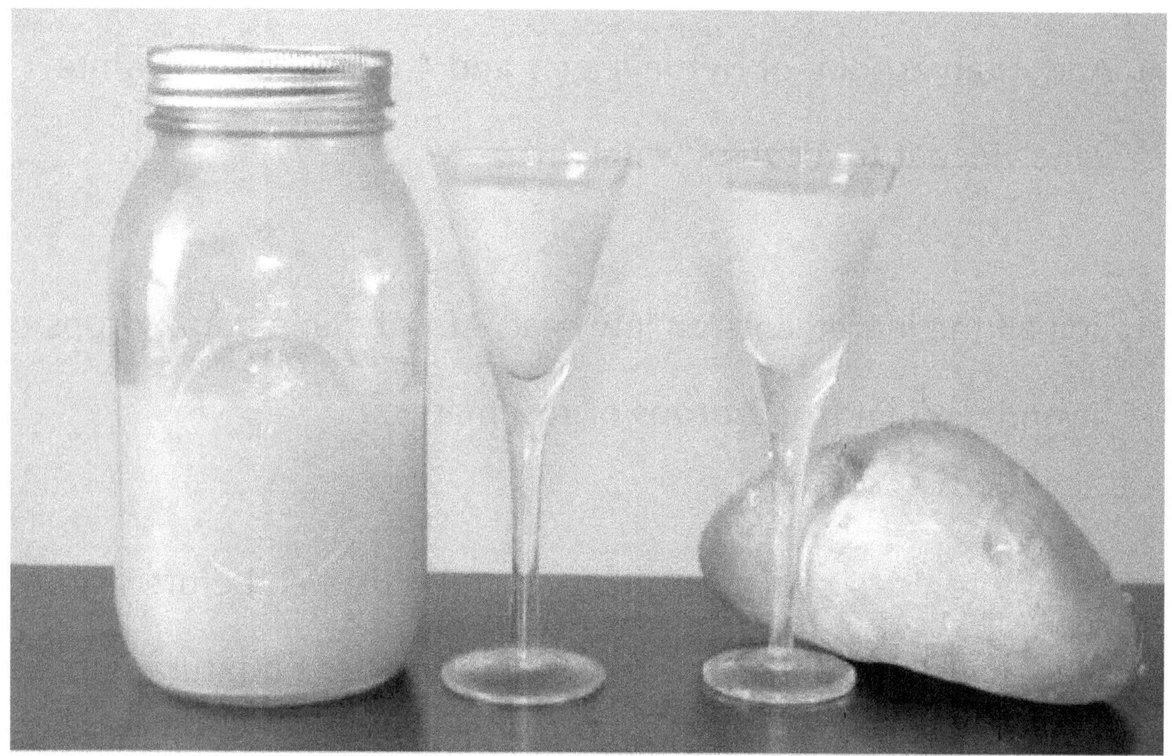

Potato juice is a surprising benefactor for hair growth.

## The Recipe:

- Wash the fresh potato well and peel off the skin, cut it into small pieces and mix them in the blender. Add some pure water in the blender, then filter.

- Apply the potato juice on your scalp and leave it on for 15 minutes.

- Potato juice is beneficial for people suffering from Alopecia and can also be used as a face pack to condition your skin.

# Aloe Vera

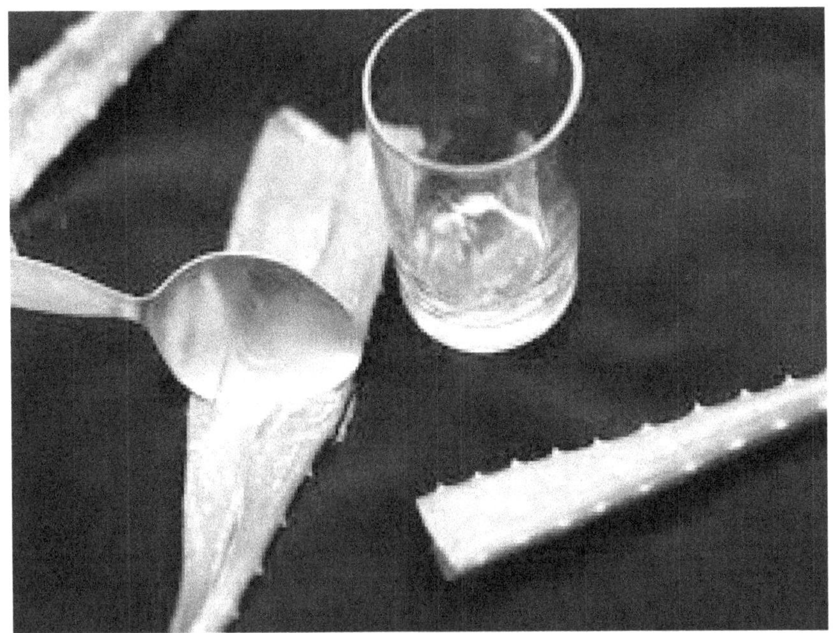

Aloe Vera gel is known for its miraculous effects on hair loss.

## The Recipe:

- Apply Aloe Vera gel and 2 tablespoon olive oil on your hair and scalp.

- Let it rest for about an hour.

- Wash off this gel gently with water and shampoo and enjoy a natural volume and shine, while giving hair growth a big boost.

# Fenugreek Recipes

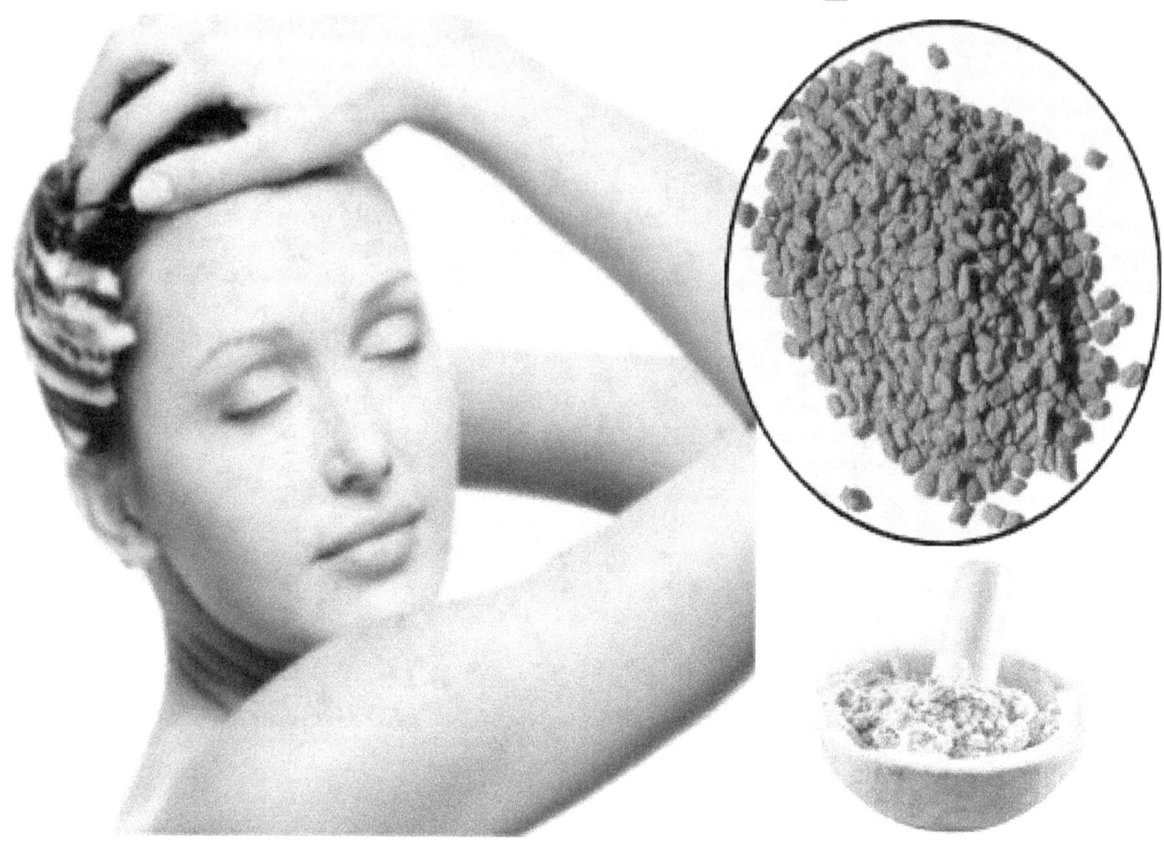

A widely used natural treatment for hair fall, fenugreek is known to protect your hair color and accelerate growth.

## The Recipe:

- Mix one teaspoon of fenugreek paste in two spoons of coconut milk and apply it on your scalp and hair.
- Leave the mixture to rest for about half an hour and wash it off.

# Another Effective Fenugreek Recipe

## The Recipe:

- Mix four tablespoons of fenugreek paste in two cloves of minced garlic and two tablespoons of olive oil.

- Add the mixture on low heat 2 minutes and apply it on your scalp.

- Then cover you hair with a plastic cap, leave the mixture to rest for about an hour and wash with shampoo.

# Apple Cider Vinegar Rinse

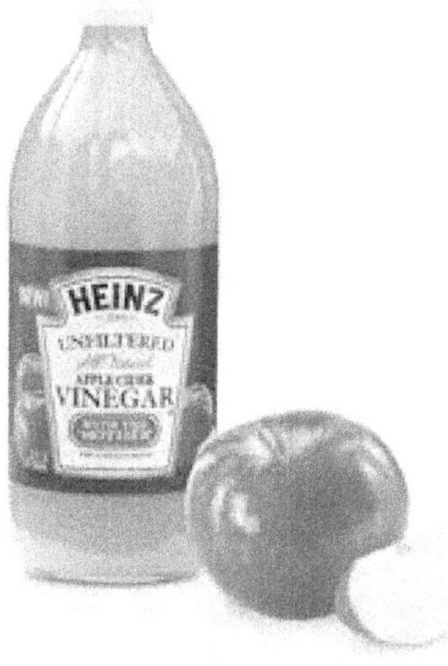

a Gentle and natural cleanser, apple cider vinegar maintains the pH balance of your hair and removes build up products from hair scalp which makes scalp easily to respire and stops hair loss. And respond to topical treatment faster.

## The Recipe:

- Mix two table spoon of apple cider vinegar to two cups of water. Rinse your scalp and hair and leave it for 15 minutes and cover it with a plastic cap.
- Then rinse well, and use your regular conditioner.
- This natural treatment is also amazing for shinier and healthier hair.
- You can use this recipe once a month or every 45 days only.

# Henna Pack

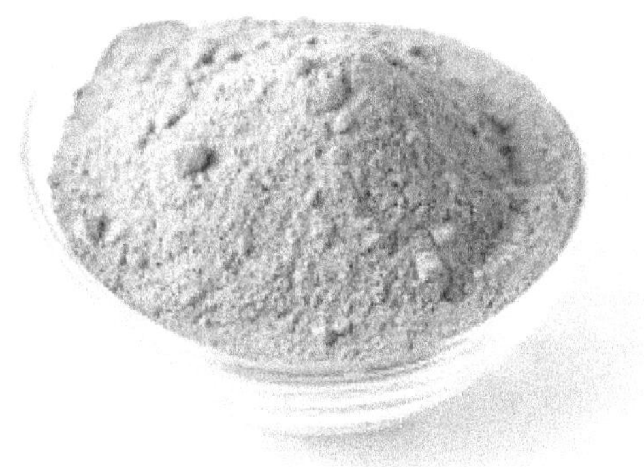

Henna is a popular hair mask, it strengthens hair roots, increases the thickness of thinning hair and cover gray hair. I recommend to use it instead of chemical hair colors at least during your hair growth journey period. It is a %100 natural treatment without any side effects.

## The Recipe:

- Mix one cup of Henna powder in small amount of yogurt or any oil and/or herbs as your choice and some warm water.
- Leave it about an hour even brewing then apply on your scalp and hair.
- Ensure to apply it to clean hair and scalp section by section.
- This mixture becomes hard as it dries. After it sets, wash it off with water and complete it with a quick shampoo wash.

Note: If you want to cover gray hair don't add oils or yogurt to henna.

# Green Tea

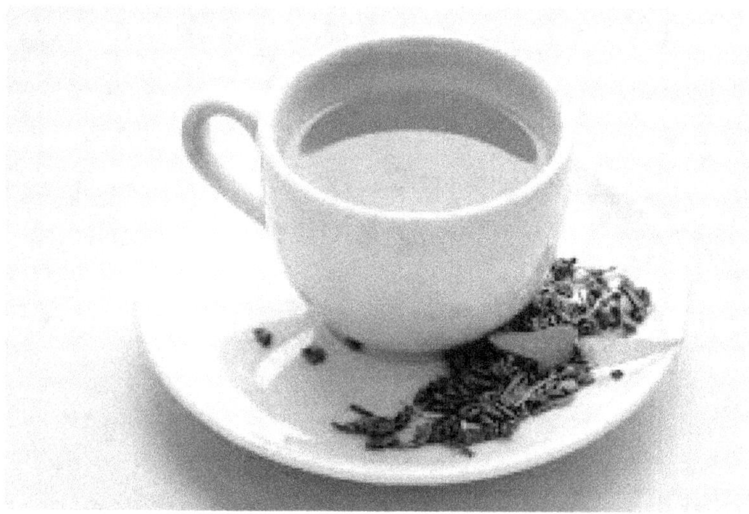

Rich in antioxidants, green tea promotes hair growth, reduces hair loss and grows hair long.

## The Recipe:

- Apply warm green tea over your scalp and hair and allow it to rest for an hour.

- Rinse it off with cool water or leave it on your hair to the next shampoo.

- Should drink one or two cups of green tea every day to improve the results. Also, you can add some peppermint paper to the tea.

# Cayenne Pepper

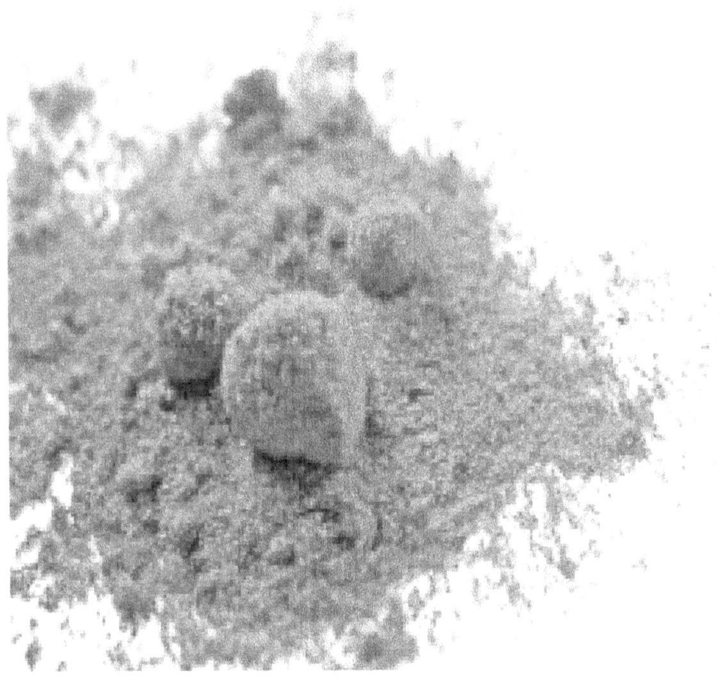

Cayenne pepper stimulates hair growth and prevents it from thinning.

## The Recipe:

- Mix a small amount of pepper powder with olive oil.

- Apply it topically on the thinning patches, leave it an hour.

- Wash it off with cool or lack warm water and use a mild shampoo.

# Rosemary

One of the most ideal hair oils is rosemary oil to prevent hair loss, it boosts cell division and expands your blood vessels in the scalp, allowing more circulation. This stimulates blood circulation, acts as a booster for hair growth.

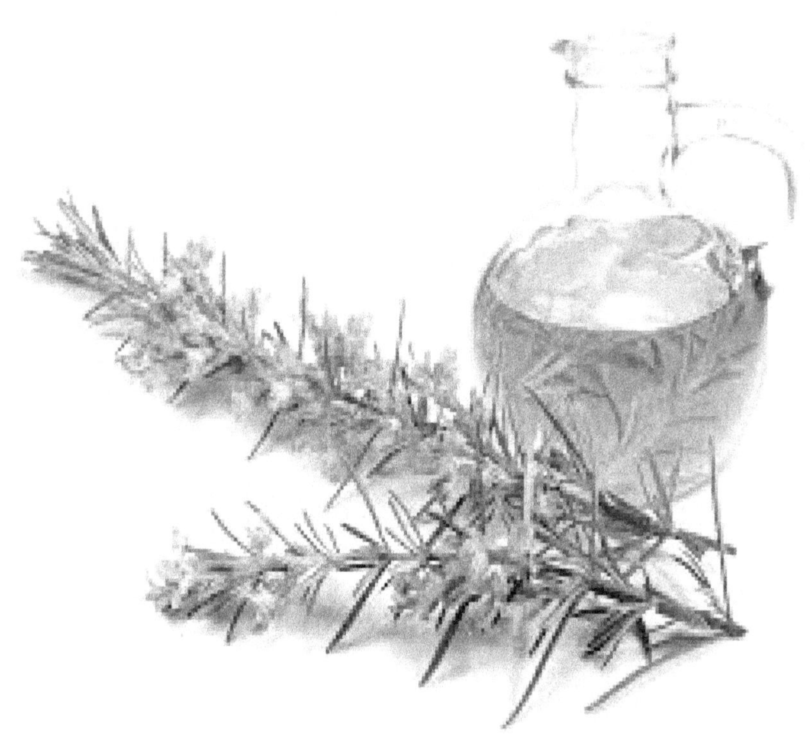

## Rosemary Oil

- Rosemary oil can be mixed with your shampoo or conditioner and also applied separately as a hair mask.

# Rosemary Leaves Tea Recipe

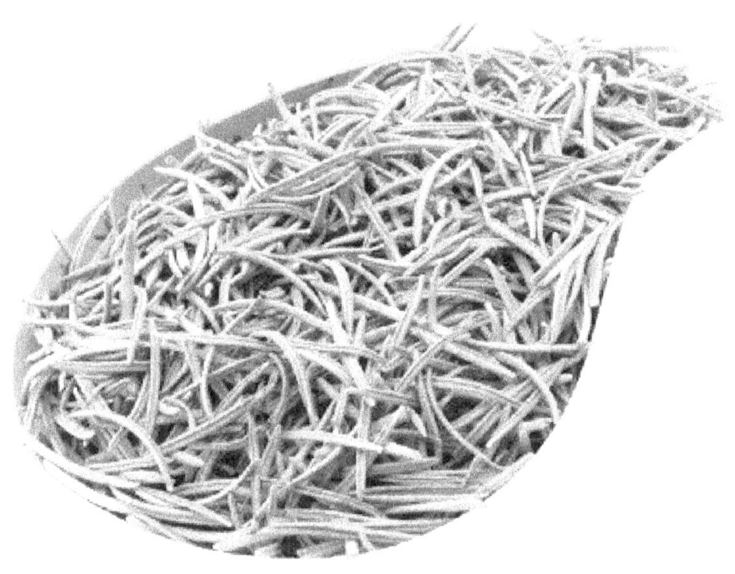

## The Recipe:

- Add 1 tablespoon of dry rosemary to a hot cup of water, after shampooing and conditioning spray your scalp with this tea, don't rinse again.

- You can add 1 tablespoon of camomile flowers with the rosemary leaves if you have dry hair.

# Sage Oil

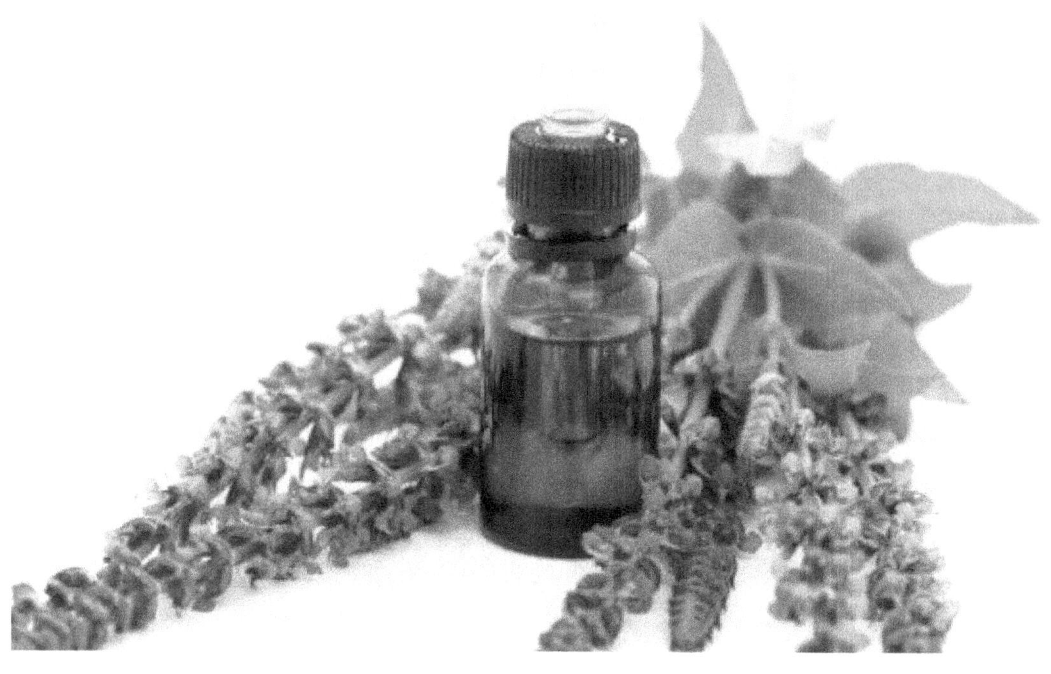

Sage oil is known for its anti hair loss and anti-acne properties and is often used to fight wrinkles and digestive problems.

## The Recipe:

- Sage oil can be combined with apple cider vinegar as a hair mask or used with other essential oils like rosemary.

- Use your fingertips to gently spread the mix onto your hair roots and massage it thoroughly.

- Allow it to settle on your scalp for about 15 minutes and wash it off.

# Lavender

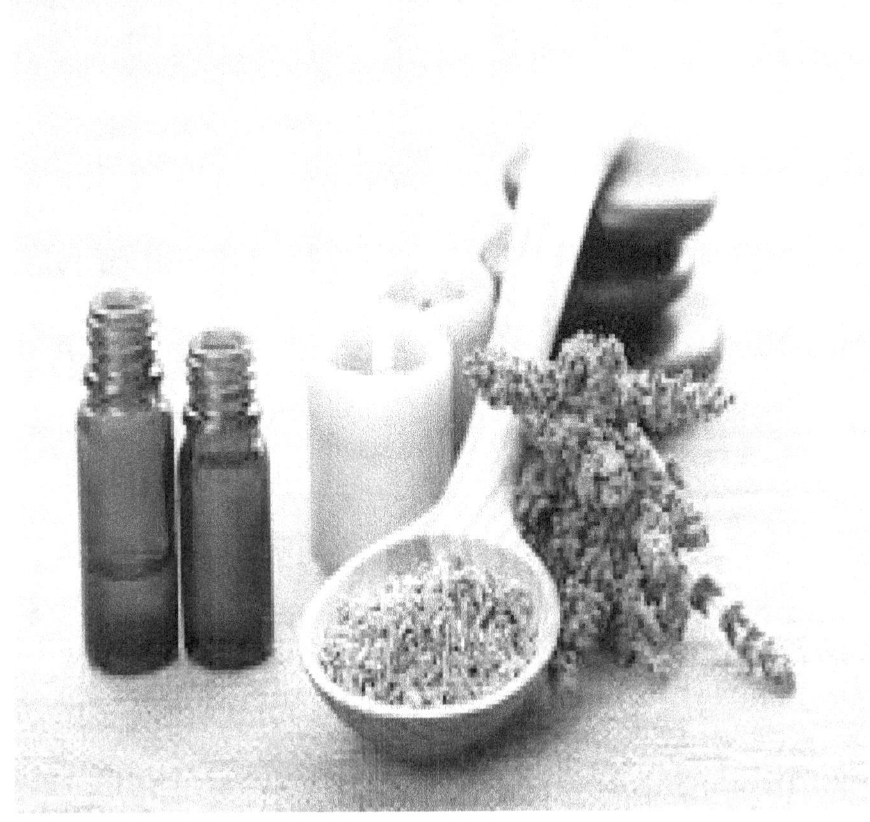

Lavender Known for its miraculous effects against hair loss patches and Alopecia, lavender oil reduces stress and improves your sleep patterns, making it a popular choice in most spa treatments.

## The Recipe:

You can prepare a complete oil mask by combining equal proportions of lavender oil, thyme oil, jojoba oil and rosemary oil and allow your scalp to absorb it for an hour. Then wash with shampoo.

# Here are Another Great Oils to Use:

## Jojoba Oil

A popular choice to moisturize and hydrate your hair, jojoba oil stimulates growth by boosting blood circulation and providing necessary moisture for follicles. It is also perfect to repair damaged and dry hair.

## Flax Seed Oil

A rich source of essential fatty acids, flax seed oil can add shine and strength to your hair. Owing to the rich reserves of omega-3 fatty acids, flax seed oil makes for an excellent supplement whether you are consuming it through diet or applying it on your hair.

## Olive Oil

Olive oil is a common ingredient in many face masks, face packs, hair tonics, scrubs and body oils owing to its natural benefits. Known to stimulate the growth of new hair, regularly using olive oil can restore your tresses and prevent the formation of the DTH hormone. Rich in antioxidants, olive oil can moisturize your scalp and make your hair smooth and silky.

# Mustard Oil

Mustard oil is rich of omega-3, this oil stimulates blood circulation, promotes hair growth and adds strength, warm it, then massage your scalp. Use it 2 to 3 times a week for best results.

# Effective Protein Masks

## Eggs Mask

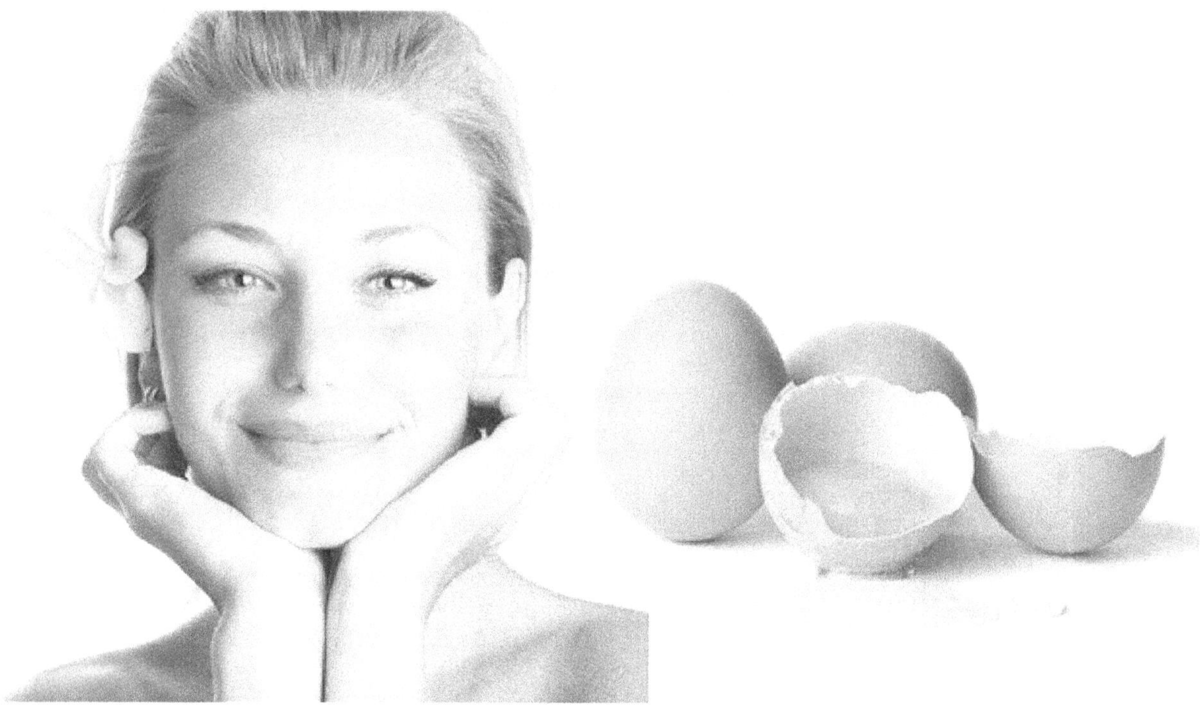

Egg is an important protein, it is the best solution when it comes to fighting hair loss, breakage and aging. Its rich protein content as well as reserves of zinc, sulfur, selenium, iron, iodine, and phosphorus make it a quick use solution.

## The Recipe:

- Mix one teaspoon of olive oil with an egg yolk to make a smooth paste. You can add honey if you have oily hair.

- Apply this paste and let it set for about 20 minutes and rinse it off with cool water and continue shampooing.

# Beef Marrow

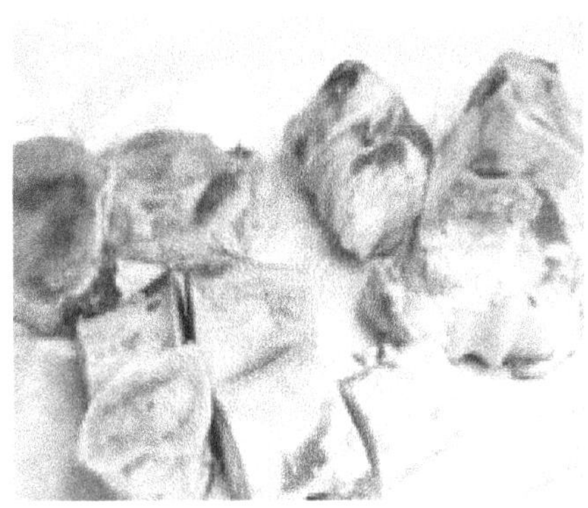

Beef marrow is rich in protein, it prevents hair loss, strengthens hair eliminates breakage completely and grows hair longer.

# The Recipe:

- Bring 5 bones with bone marrow from the butcher, remove the marrow from the bones, then boil on low heat until the marrow melts and become like oil, leave it to cool, then apply it to hair and scalp.

- Cover with a plastic cap, leave it about 30 to 60 minutes, then wash very well with **Clarifying Shampoo** because this mask is very thick.

# Coconut Milk

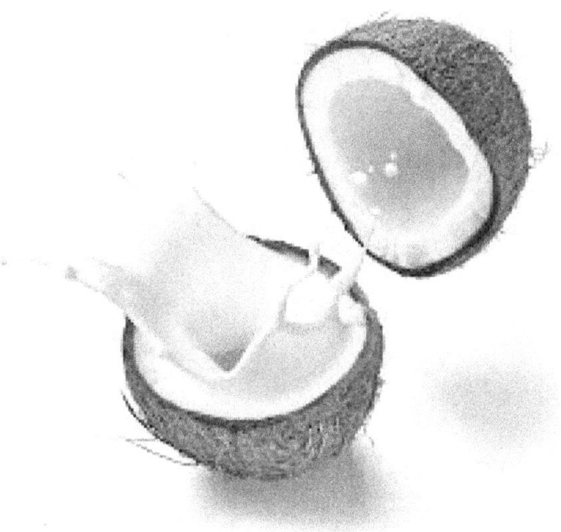

Coconut is rich in essential fats, protein, potassium, Vitamin C and iron, coconut milk can reduce hair shedding and breakage.

## The Recipe:

Use coconut milk extract and apply it on hair and scalp. Allow it to work its magic overnight and rinse it off with water the next morning.

**Warning:** Do not use any protein mask more than one time every 15 days, as applying protein too much damages hair.

# How to Make
# Faster Hair Growth Shampoo

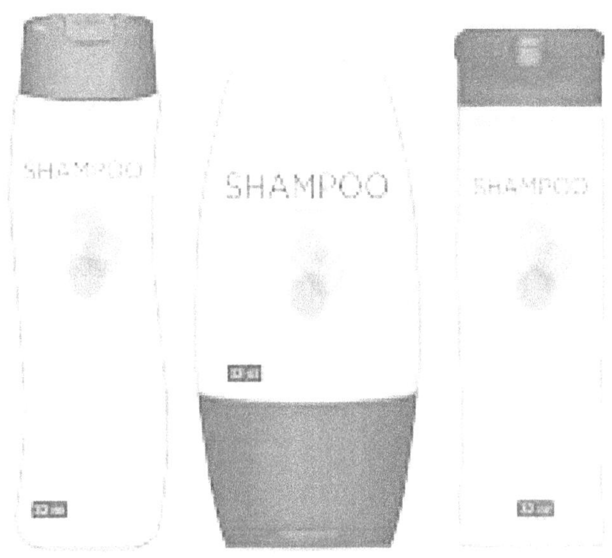

If you are serious about reversing the damage caused to your hair, you can start by improving your shampoo. Instead of blindly depending on store bought products, you can make effective and natural shampoo at home. There are many benefits provided by a homemade shampoo as it can accelerate hair growth and reduce hair loss. This particular homemade shampoo is rich in vitamins and minerals including sulfur, zinc, vitamin B and C, nourishing your hair, promoting and prolonging the Anagen phase of hair growth.

# Ingredients:

- 250 ml shampoo

- 1/2 onion

- 2 or 3 large cloves of garlic

- Jojoba oil –(optional)

- Blender

- Gauze

# The Recipe:

- Start by choosing the right shampoo that suits your hair type. As far as possible, stick to organic shampoos that don't contain artificial preservatives and sulfates that provide lather. If you have dandruff, choose honey based shampoos.

- Cut the garlic and onions before adding it in the shampoo to very small cubes. While the onion helps condition and strengthens your hair, the garlic serves as an anti-fungal and anti-bacterial element.

- You can also use a few drops of jojoba oil if needed as it fights scalp infections and impurities.

- Start by adding the garlic and onion mix to the shampoo in a container and leave it in the fridge for about 3-4 days.

- After it has settled in the shampoo, use the shampoo like any shampoo, or you can transfer the contents to a blender and thoroughly mix the ingredients together.

- Filter it using the gauze before using the shampoo.

- This homemade shampoo works best when used 2-3 times a week.

- Start by wetting your hair and applying small amounts of shampoo and massage your scalp thoroughly. After shampooing, resume using your hair conditioner and mask.

# Important Notes:

- ➥ Ensure that you shake the bottle before using the shampoo for even distribution.

- ➥ Always store the homemade shampoo in the refrigerator after every use to preserve it contents.

- ➥ If your scalp is particularly sensitive or itchy, avoid using the garlic and stick to just jojoba oil and onion.

- ➥ It is not necessary to blend the ingredients by the blender.

## Use This Shampoo After Using Your Ordinary Shampoo.

# Modern Hair Loss Treatments

## Laser Therapy

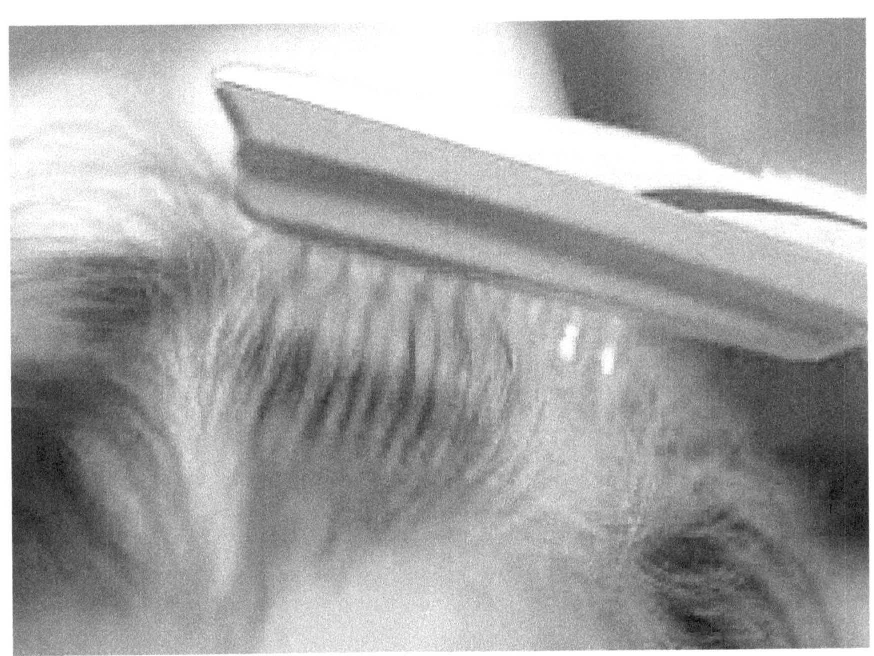

Known commonly as low dose laser therapy, this treatment is used to tackle hair loss caused by genetics. Pattern balding or Alopecia in men and women can be treated with this method, also known as red light therapy, soft laser, cold laser,photobiomodulation and biostimulation. Since the balding patterns of men and women are fairly unique, laser therapy can be attuned to treat different cases.

Carefully, the most popular laser therapies for pattern balding include hair transplants, finasteride and minoxidil.

Low light laser therapy works by increasing blood flow and circulation in your scalp and stimulating your hair follicles.

These results in more strands of hair reaching the Anagen phase instead of the Telogen phase.

➡ The Best Laser Hair Therapy is low level laser therapy message helmet, because it contains laser and massage at the same time.

**Please Visit http://fasterhair.net/laserhelmet for More Details!**

# Scalp Injections

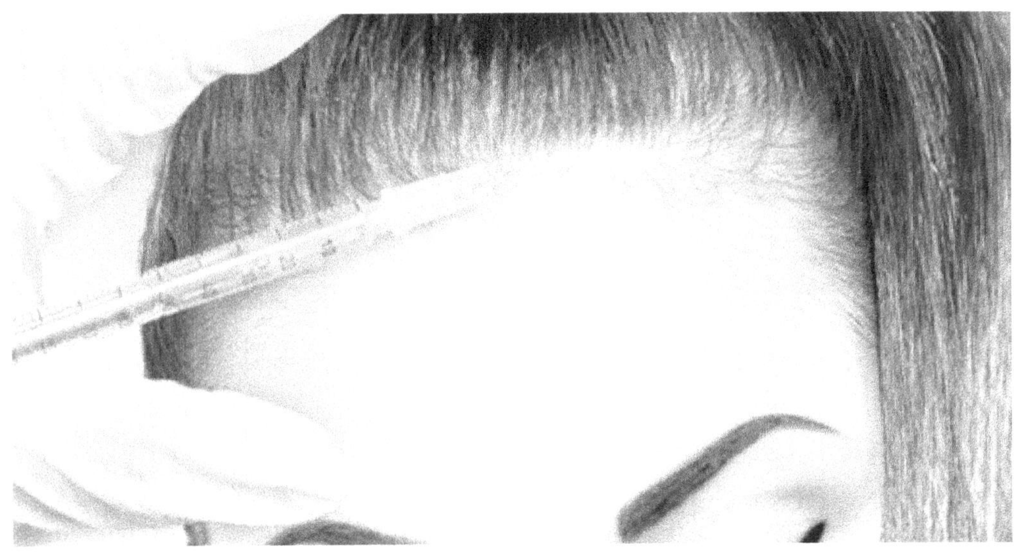

## Cortisone Injections

One of the most popular scalp injections administered to treat hair loss include cortisone injections.

Containing anti-inflammatory medication, cortisone injections are ideal to treat alopecia areata, pseudopelade, traction alopecia, Telogen effluvium, pattern baldness and Trichotillomania.

Each case includes cortisone injections numbering between two and 50 depending on the size of the balding area and the severity of the hair loss.

# Mesotherapy Injections

Mesotherapy is a fairly less invasive hair growth procedure that is also completed in very less time.

This procedure rarely takes over 30 minutes to finish and includes one sitting. During the treatment, the middle layer of the skin known as mesoderm is stimulated via injections that contain a unique combination of minerals, vitamins, homeopathic medicines and traditional pharmaceuticals.

The concentration of the injection fluid is mainly based on the severity of the case and can take anywhere between four and 15 sittings, over a period of 1-2 weeks.

Since the injections are directly administered to the target skin layer, very little medication is required to bring noticeable results. Unlike most other surgical procedures, you can avoid a wide range of side effects by opting for Mesotherapy.

# Plasma Injections

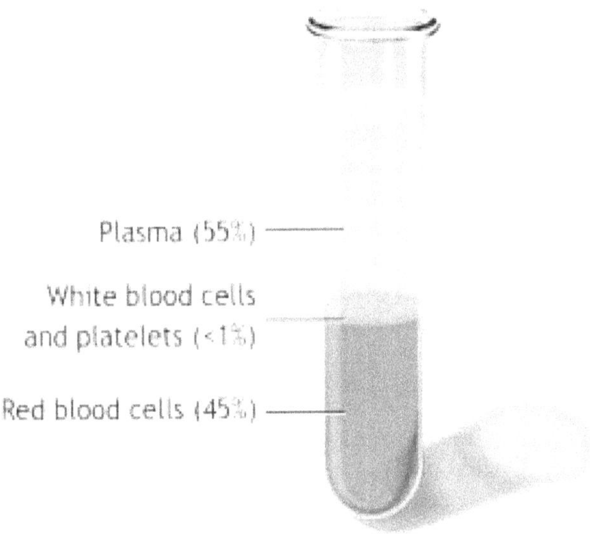



Plasma injections, also known as platelet rich plasma is counted amongst the most effective treatment options for hair loss. It is the newest hair growth technique.

This simple clinical procedure is very safe and is usually administered by a licensed dermatologist. Also known as PRP, this therapy has the same effects as that of a vampire facelift that helps build collagen and reduces lines and scars.

This procedure involves centrifuging the blood in your scalp and collecting the plasma in a tube. The platelets rich in plasma are essential for healing and tissue regeneration.

This plasma is then injected or rubbed onto your scalp. The entire treatment lasts about eight sitting, with a two-week gap between each session. Hair loss medication like minoxidil or propercia is also prescribed along with it.

PRP is an ideal option for men and women experiencing alopecia or a receding hairline for any reason.

People with pattern baldness can also benefit from platelet rich plasma injections. While the treatment yields excellent results for most people, it is not recommended for people who have already lost all their hair.

Plasma injections strengthens, thicken existing hair and help growing new hair on a bald patch. it has zero side effects as it is already from your body and i recommend it.

- Here are 2 good youtube videos you can watch to learn how this scalp injection works:

Dr.Thomas Barnes' PRP Hair Growth

Dr. Joseph Greco - Using PRP Therapy For Hair Loss

# Try these Amazing Tricks!

Here are some amazing ideas to try that can help you hide thinning hair and bald areas until your hair grow again:

## Microfiber Keratin

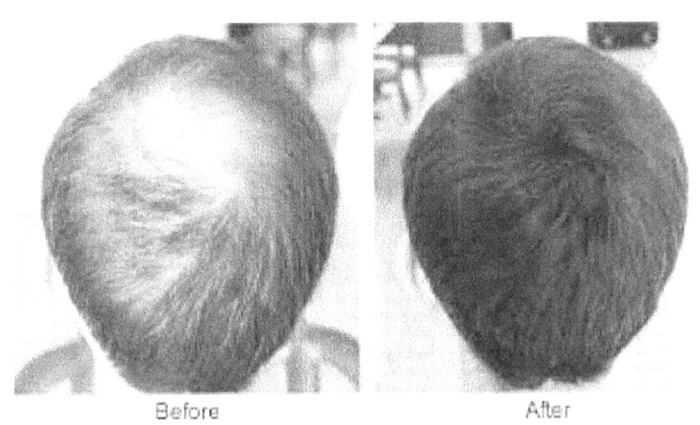



Keratin fibers commercially available are made from the same organic protein as your hair. These fibers are charged with limited amounts of electrostatic energy that allow them to intertwine with your original hair. Made purely of protein, keratin fibers do not contain chemicals or additives and have no side effects. Moreover, they are one of the fastest ways to improve your appearance and deal with thinning hair on your scalp. They neither promote nor interfere with hair growth and pose as a quick fix to give your tresses a thicker and fuller appearance.

Keratin fibers are compatible with your scalp even when you are undergoing other hair loss treatments and are available in several colors to seamlessly blend with your natural hair or colored hair.

High quality keratin fibers are completely natural and do not stain. Keratin fibers can also be customized to your hair texture and blend with short, long, straight, curly and dyed hair.

Binding with your hair, keratin fibers are sweat resistant, water resistant, stain resistant and do not easily peel off.
Keratin fibers are usually available in spray cans and can be easily applied on your scalp.

Owing to the safe and hassle free application, keratin fibers can be applied in your home and do not require the assistance of professionals in a salon or clinic, making it a preferred and highly affordable solution to deal with hair loss.

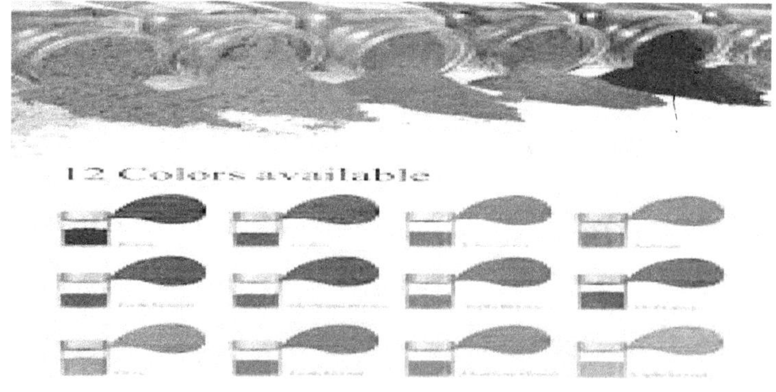

# Volume Products

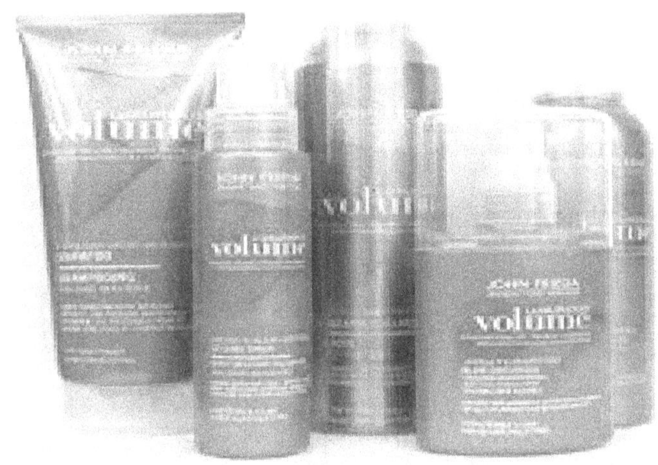

Volume products are also ideal for thinning, fine, weightless and flat hair, try to use it to add volume and double your hair weight and size in a minute. These products are usually available in the form shampoo, conditioner, powder, mask and spray. I tried an inexpensive volume shampoo and conditioner called <u>Luxurious volume by John Frieda</u> it worked well. Another amazing <u>volume products are from Redken</u>. But it should be after using any volume shampoo and/or conditioner to apply some moisturiser as these kinds of shampoos for some people may cause dryness.

# Back Comb

Another great idea for thin hair is backcombing to create a puffing look, the back combing adds volume and weight, to do this; Simply section your hair to small parts, then start to back combing each part with soft brush or comb. Look the image.

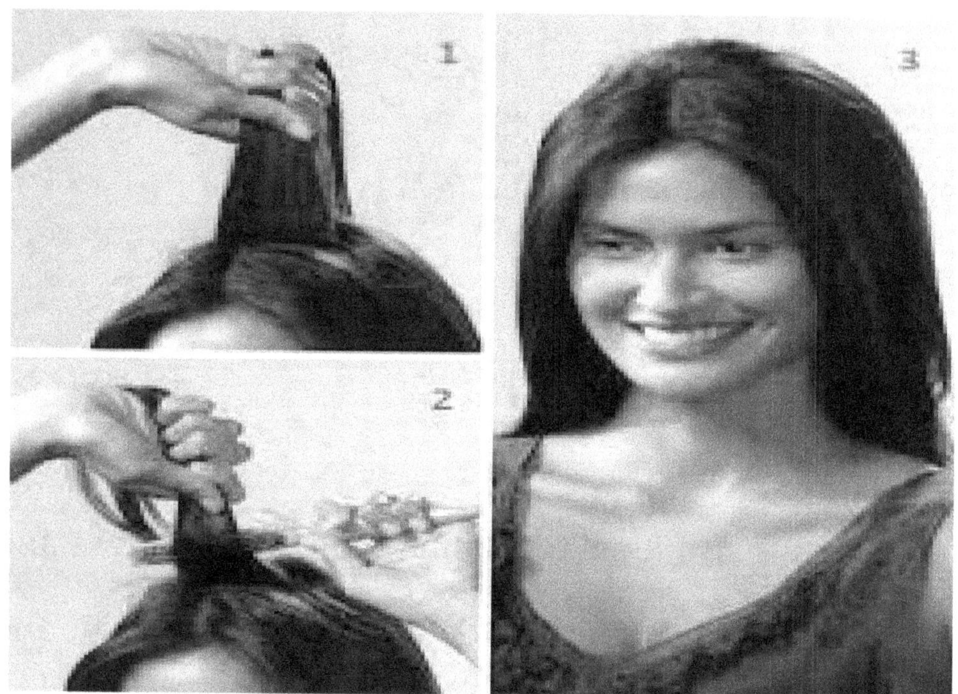

Back Comb

# Dark Hair Colors

If you have thin hair with light color, try to darken your hair color with dark shades like medium brown, dark brown or black. Dark colors add volume and make hair look healthy. You can use natural Henna to get the dark color.

# Exercises to Promote Hair Growth

Through regular stretching and physical exertion, you can prevent the buildup of acid in your muscles and remain limber and strong. This will help you maintain healthier and stronger hair. By improving blood circulation through exercise, you are providing fresh oxygen and nutrients to your hair cells.

Working out is also a great solution for stress relief. You may already know by now that stress is not good for your hair, making exercise a great pastime to relax, unwind and strengthen yourself. By keeping your stress levels in check and giving yourself a regular fix of an endorphin rush, you will not only enjoy a better mood and lower stress, but will also get thicker tresses.

Any exercise that involves inverted poses or back-bends is known to help hair growth. By increasing the blood flow and circulation to your scalp, you are relieving tension from your neck and back muscles and slowing down hair loss.

# Back-Bends

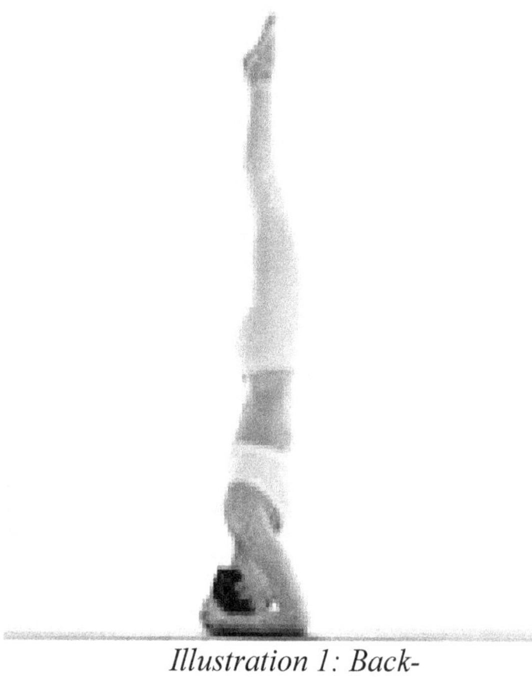

*Illustration 1: Back-Bends*

Apart from engaging in <u>yoga</u>, cardio and going for a jog, you can engage in specialized exercises for your scalp. These exercises can range from a simple head massage to a full blown hour long session to become fitter and stronger. Headstands and a balanced cardio session can work wonders in circulating blood in your scalp and improving the condition of your hair. Apart from these, you can also follow these <u>yoga exercises</u>.

    136

# Inverted Poses Yoga

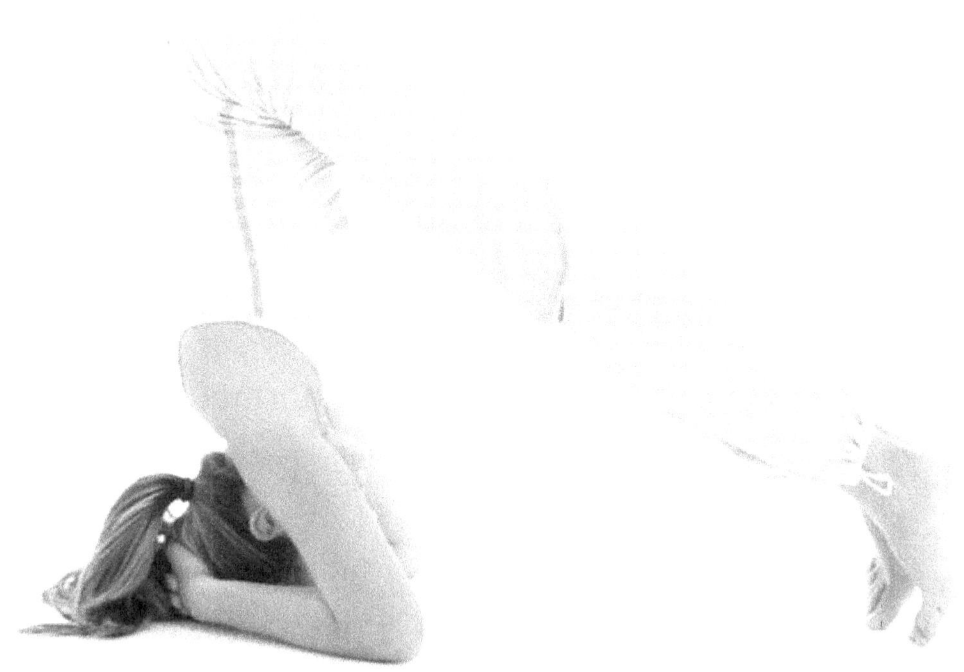

*Illustration 2: inverted poses yoga*

# Triangle Pose (Trikonasana)

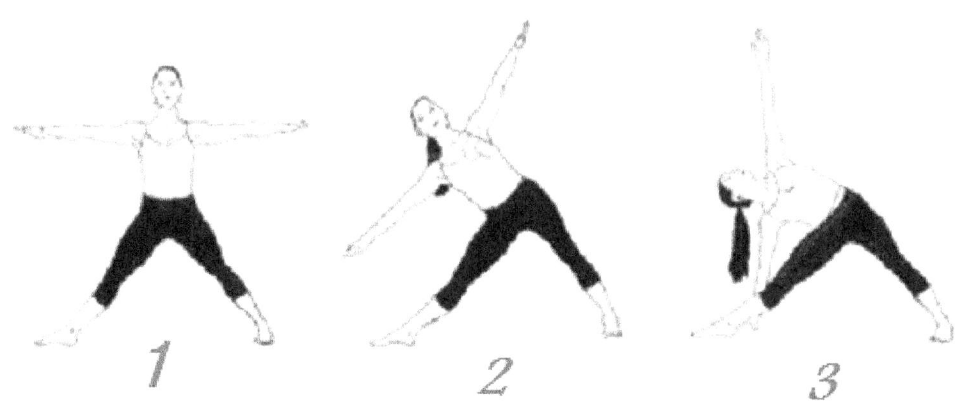


*Illustration 3: Triangle Pose*

Stand erect with your feet placed three feet apart. Raise both your hands to shoulder level and maintain this position while breathing normally. Bend to your right and touch the toes of your feet with the fingers of your right hand.

You can also attempt a cross triangle pose by touching your left hand fingers to your right foot. Hold that position for at least 30 seconds, or longer if possible. Raise your hands to the normal position and perform the same step on the right side.

# Fish pose (Matsyasana)

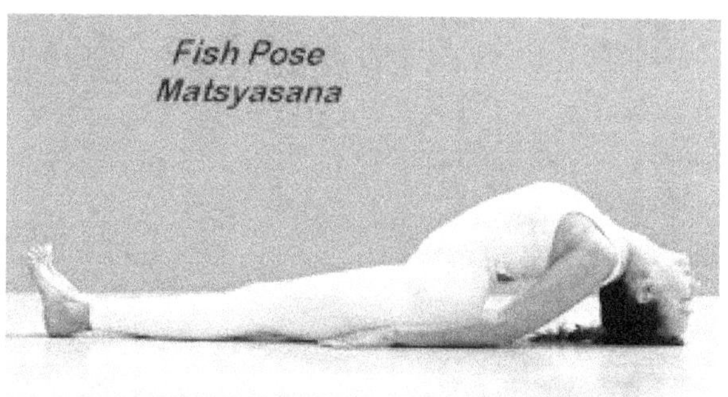


*Illustration 4: Fish pose (Matsyasana)*

This simple yet effective exercise works wonders by improving circulation in your scalp. Start by lying on your back and keep your hands next to your thighs, palms facing down. Slide your hands beneath your buttocks and a take a deep breath, while lifting your head and chest. Ensure that your buttocks are on the ground the entire time and drop your head back such that you are resting on your crown. Rest your torso on your elbows and crown and maintain this position for as long as possible. Straighten your head slowly and carefully and release yourself from this position. Repeat these steps a few times during each exercise session for best results.

# Plough Pose (Halasana)

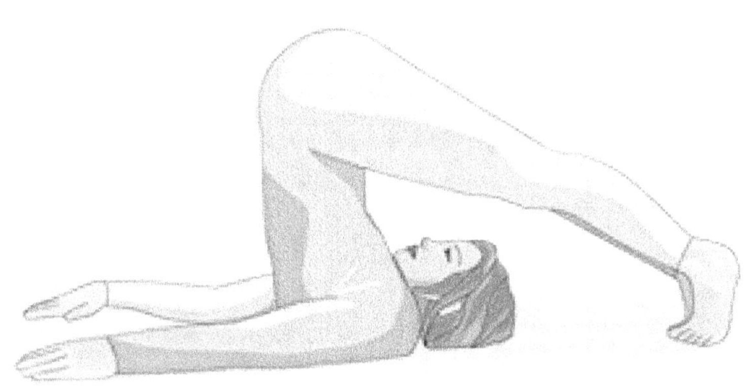

*Illustration 5: Plough pose or Plow Pose (Halasana)*

Start this exercise by lying flat on your back on a comfortable mat. Place your hands facing downwards comfortably by your sides. Slowly lift your legs and keep them at a right angle to the floor. Maintain this position for a few seconds and continue lifting your legs further until they reach over your head and touch the ground behind. Once you have stabilized this position, touch your chin against the throat and

retain this position without moving your hands. Breathe normally and

deeply and return to your original position slowly. Repeat this step a

few times.

# Knee to Chest Pose (Apanasana)

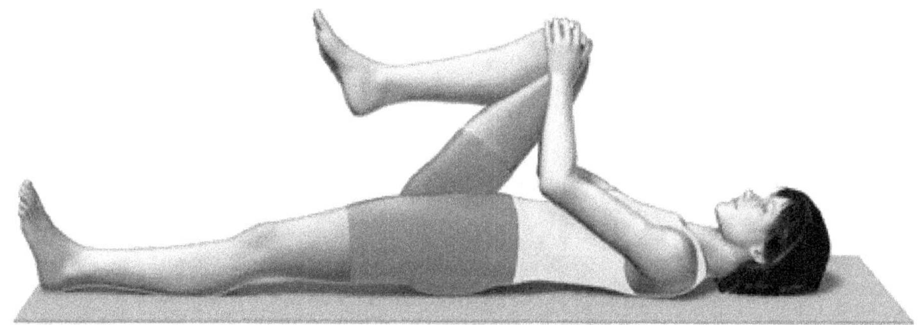

*Illustration 6: Knee to chest pose 1*

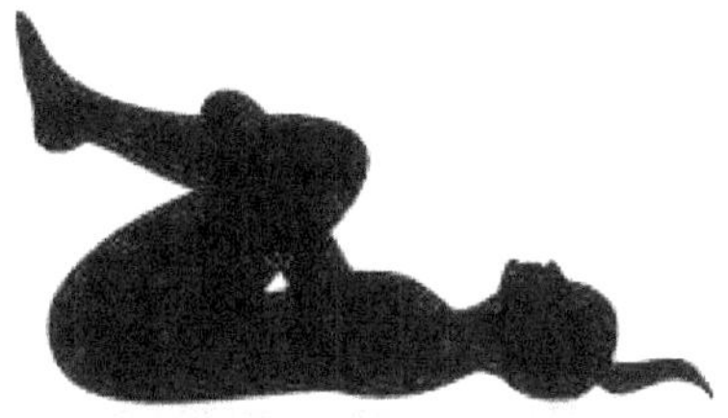



Lie flat on your back. Start this exercise by folding your legs at the knees and bring them closer to your chest. Use your palms to hold the knee caps and ensure that your fingers face your feet. Inhale deeply and slowly, while straightening your arms and push the legs slightly away from its current position.

After a few seconds, exhale and bring your legs closer to your chest. Continue this pattern for a few minutes or for as long as you are comfortable.

When you are done, slowly move your legs away from your body and perform a side twist with your folded knees – once to your left and once to the right. Straighten your legs and place your palms facing down to your side.

    

# Detox for Healthy Hair

Your hair goes through a lot of trauma in a single day, apart from battling the increasing pollution to handling poor diets, chemical bleaches and color. It comes as no surprise when you realize that your hair needs a drastic detox. If you have subjected your hair to regular chemical colors, hot irons and other heat styling appliances, it is time to give it a gentle and nourishing experience. Apart from the pollution and the styling nightmares, your hair also faces significant damage caused by exposure to heat and sun. With regular exposure to the harsh sunlight and UV rays, your tresses regularly need a thorough detoxification, just like your body.

It is not enough to simply take care of your hair, but you must also detoxify your body. After all, everything you eat and are exposed to has a direct effect on the state of your hair. If you want to better your hair, the detoxification should begin from the core i.e. your body. The following steps can guide you in making a home detox system for your tired hair.

# Quick Detox for Your Body

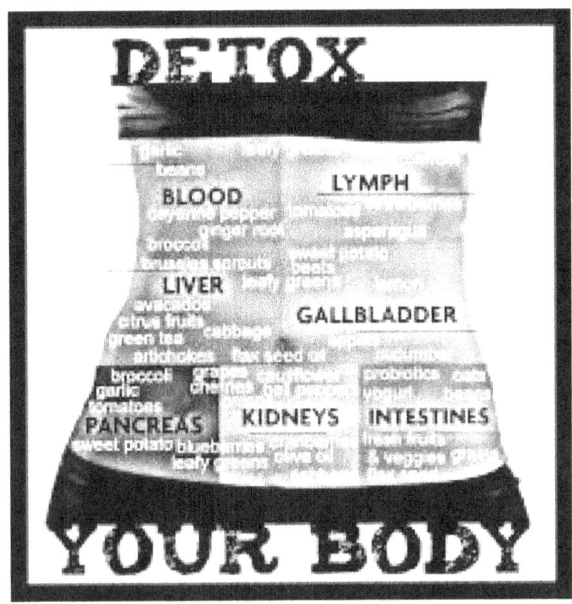


By removing chemicals and harmful toxins from your body, you can make your hair detox even more effective. It is important to remember that your energy levels may fall during the course of the detox. That is why it is best to schedule it on a day off or at the beginning of your weekend. Start your detox on the first night of the weekend and avoid going to work or performing strenuous tasks. It is also a good idea to remain relaxed throughout the weekend and avoid going to places that require high amounts of energy. This includes partying at a club or engaging in binge drinking. The whole point of the detox is to rid your body of undesirable elements.

For the first dinner of the detox, start with a green salad with a delicious vinaigrette dressing. Ensure that you eat a healthy portion of the salad. Do not starve yourself. Drink a full glass of water before you go to sleep. In the morning, take a dose of vitamin C supplement. To remain safe, get the right supplement and dosage from your GP. Have a tall glass of organic fruit juice for breakfast. Avoid drinking juice from a packaged product or concentrate. Do not put extra sugar or sweeteners in the juice and steer clear of products that contain HFCS.

If possible, dice up your favorite fruit and blend a fruit juice at home. You can make juices of different fruits to keep it interesting and drink one glass every two hours. Always carry enough water and drink a few sips when you feel hungry. Ensure that you drink at least eight glasses of water a day to remain hydrated. For dinner, have a full bowl of brown rice or broth. Repeat the same process for another day. During your detox, it is best to stay away from drinking or smoking as it completely defeats the purpose. While your body is detoxifying, prepare to detox your hair.

# Clean Your Colon for Better Hair

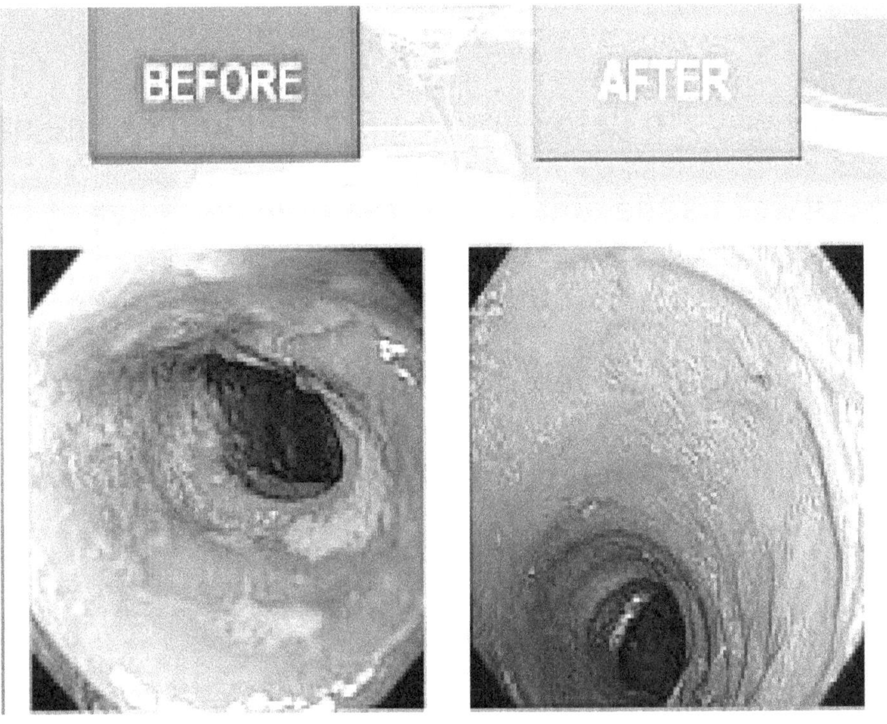


Colon stores dirt and toxins which cause weak health, hair loss and slow growing. Colon Cleansing is one of the best methods you can do to stop hair loss and improve your health. By removing dirt and toxins from your colon, your hair will stop falling. People who have done this method noticed a big changes in their hair health.

To clean your colon simply pay a visit to a doctor ask him to clean your colon or you can clean the colon at home by Enema.

# How to Detox Your Hair
## "Multiple methods"

There are many ways to detox your hair depending on the natural ingredients as well as the amount of free time you have at hand. Don't forget to play some relaxing music in the background or light calming incense to soothe your nerves. This stage is all about relaxation and purification; creating a calm and peaceful environment is equally important.

# Method 1: Clay Shampoo

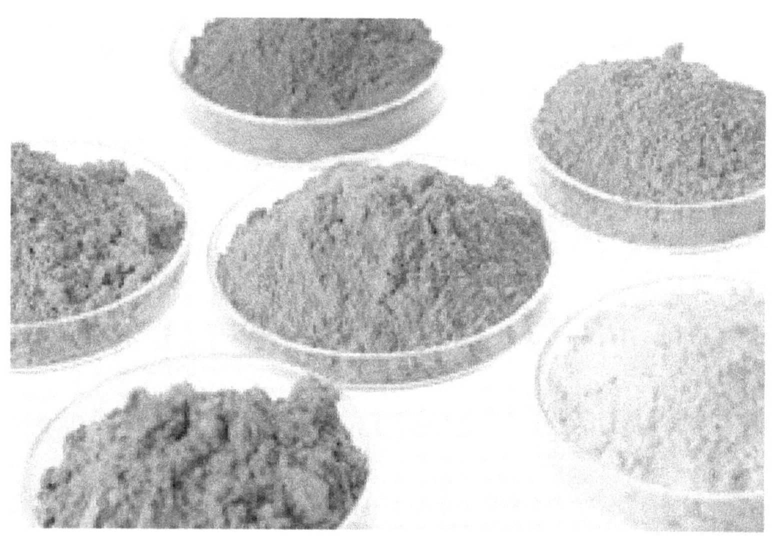

This quick method will help you cleanse and purify your hair with simple day to day ingredients available at home or the local supermarket.

Start this short method by rinsing your hair with water in the sink, enough to wet it completely. You can wrap a towel around your shoulders to ensure that your clothes don't get wet.

Squeeze a normal amount of organic or chemical-free shampoo in your palm and mix it with an equal amount of clay facial mask. You can also choose any other clay-based cleansing product that is ideal for your skin.

Mix them thoroughly and run it through your hair, ensuring that you cover your hair with this mix from the root to the tip. You can vary the amount of shampoo and clay mask depending on the length of your hair.

Allow the mask to relax in your hair for about five minutes. While the shampoo removes silicates from previous washes, the clay mask removes impurities. After the mask has set, rinse it off thoroughly and gently dry your hair by patting it. It is best to allow your hair to dry naturally.

# Method 2: Baking Soda Shampoo

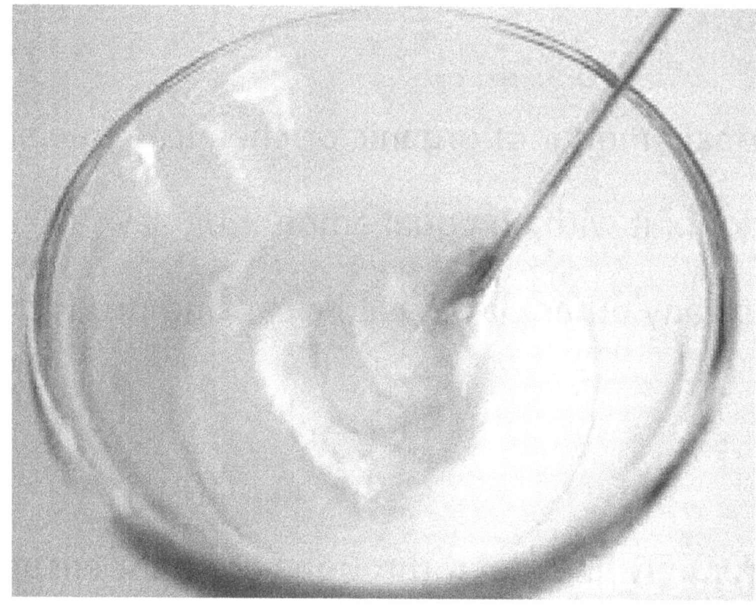

Before you begin, ensure that you have your ingredients ready for use. Start by making yourself relaxed and comfortable. This method is carried out in three stages, starting with a thorough cleansing treatment. Clean your hair and scalp by mixing about quarter a cup of baking soda in three cups of hot water. This water should be as hot as possible without burning your skin or hair. Wet your hair thoroughly and pour this mixture while massaging your scalp and hair thoroughly. Let the mixture sit for a few minutes before you rinse it off.

# Method 3: Lemon Juice

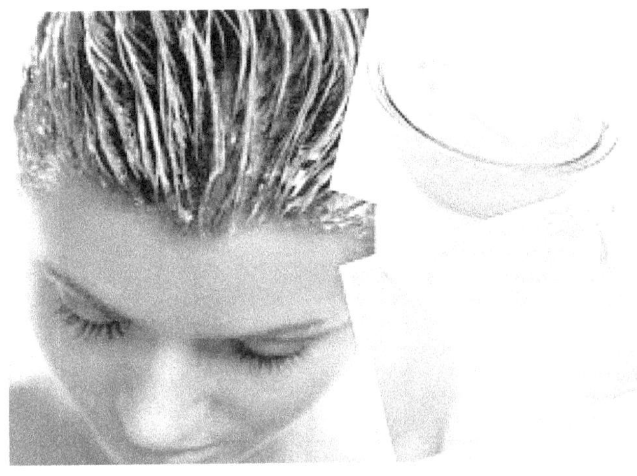

If your hair is damaged and undernourished, it is important to bring back its strength with the right natural ingredients. This simple homemade concoction will help you nurse your hair back to life. Combine an egg with one tablespoon of fresh lemon juice, one teaspoon of apple cider vinegar and about two tablespoons of any hair oil. You can use olive oil, coconut oil, sunflower oil, avocado oil or any other oil. Blend the ingredients thoroughly in a mixer a few times. Wet your hair thoroughly and pour this mixture onto your hair, massaging your scalp and tresses. Pay special attention to your tired roots and spread the mixture over your scalp thoroughly. Allow this mixture to rest in your hair for about two minutes and wash it off with warm water.

>> You can also make a lemon rinse for oily hair and scalp, that by mix 2 tablespoons lemon juice and 4 cups of lack-warm water and rinse your hair after shampoo and conditioner. Don't rinse again.

# Method 4: Hot Oil Treatment

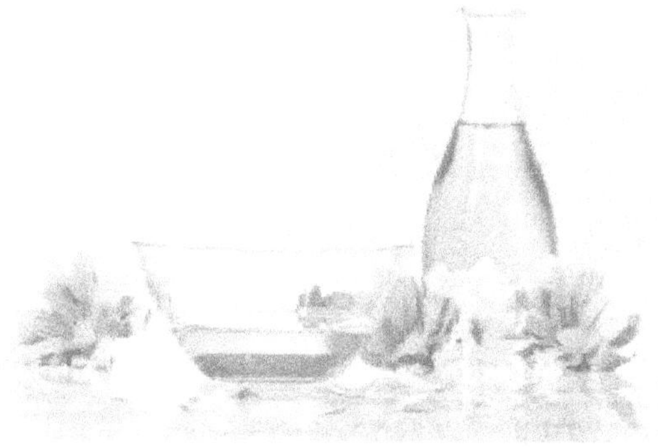

a Homemade hot oil treatment is a great way to repair damage caused by pollutants, smoke and dust. Combine 1/4 cup of almond oil, sunflower oil, avocado oil or olive oil. Store this mixture in a glass container and if you have very long hair, double the quantity of all ingredients used in the recipe. In a pan, boil some water and place the container in the pan to heat up the contents. Allow the contents to cool down if it gets too hot. Remember, the ingredients should be warm, but not so hot that it burns your skin or hair.

Dampen your hair slightly and apply the mixture from roots to the damaged ends. Cover your hair with a shower cap or use a hair steamer and enjoy a warm shower for a few minutes. This heats up your scalp and hair without washing away the hot oil mixture. After 15-20 minutes, rinse it off your hair with a gentle shampoo.

# Simple Tips to Maintain Healthy Hair

Long, thick and lustrous hair is something that requires a lot of time, care and patience. While it was possible to enjoy luxurious locks in the past, the fast paced lifestyles today don't allow much room for this. If you are a busy, modern woman, adhering to the practices of the past for hair care may not always be possible. That is the reason why you should make the best of the situation. The following tips are practical, simple and effective. By following these simple tips regularly, you will see a noticeable improvement in the texture, strength and shine of your hair.

## Brushing Your Hair the Right Way

Brushing your hair the right way plays an important role in maintaining healthy hair. The old wives' tale of brushing your hair 100 times every night has some merit. In fact, the practice is very beneficial to your hair as it helps distribute natural oils evenly along the roots and the tips. With a quality hair brush, you can make your hair shinier, stronger and less prone to breakage. This practice can also help you eliminate some hair care products and keep your locks naturally healthy. Start by brushing your hair at the bottom and work your way up to tangle gently. After you have smoothed your hair, you can smoothly brush it from root to tip.

It is ideal to use a boar bristle brush. Although they are slightly expensive than regular brushes, they are beneficial and long lasting. The dense construction of the hairbrush allows you to remove debris, dirt and dust from your hair and keep it clean.

The bristles on these brushes are tough and flexible and can be used for all hair textures including curly and unmanageable hair. It is best not to brush your hair when wet as the roots will be weak.

After your hair has dried sufficiently, use a wide toothed comb to tangles. It is also important to remember not to brush your hair too often. While regular combing and brushing stimulates the hair follicles, brushing or combing too often can lead to frizzing, split ends and damage.

# Police Your Shampoos and Conditioners

Washing your hair regularly helps keep it clean. However, there are many who overdo it and end up damaging their hair. Washing your hair too often can remove the natural oils found in the hair and leave it dry and damaged. It is best to wash your hair twice a week with a high quality, chemical-free shampoo. Choose shampoos that do not contain sulfates as they can damage your hair.

These chemicals are mainly incorporated to make your shampoo lather up while other preservatives like parabens can cause irritation in your eyes. These chemicals are neither good for your hair nor the environment. It is also important to choose a shampoo that is geared towards your hair texture and type.

Coarse or curly hair is best cleaned with anti-frizz or softening shampoos while dry hair requires shampoos with more collagen and glycerin. Similarly, oily hair is best cleaned with gentle daily use shampoos and colored or salon treated hair is best nourished with shampoos fortified with amino acids and protein extracts.

Apply the same rules on your conditioner and make a choice based on your hair type, damage, and length. Different conditioners are ideal for thick hair when compared to finer hair.

It is also important to avoid using products with too much protein as they can make your hair brittle.

# Trim Your Locks Regularly

Perfect hair also means getting rid of split ends regularly. If your hair has started resembling an old paint brush, it is time to cut short those locks and get rid of split ends. You don't have to invest a lot of time and money by visiting a salon simply to get a trim. If you do not wish to cut your hair too short, you can trim your hair yourself at home with a mirror and a pair of scissors.

# Leave Your Hair Natural

While the demand for hair colors and artificial dyes increase every day, many are realizing their ill-effects. As much as possible, avoid dyeing your hair. Hair that has been treated in the salon for perming, straightening, streaks or coloring often face more damage as they are exposed to heat and chemicals. On the other hand, women who choose to show off their natural hair  rarely experience the damage and dryness caused by chemical processing. Even if you do wish to dye your hair, do it sparingly and choose quality hair colors.

# Go Easy on the Styling

It is important to note that styling your hair occasionally will not have any adverse effects on your hair. However, if you expose your hair to heat and other styling appliances multiple times a week, your hair will experience damage. As much as possible, avoid perming, curling, straightening, crimping or bleaching your hair altogether. While it is alright to straighten or curl your hair for a special occasion, it is best done sparingly.

Avoid using rubber bands to pull back or style your hair as they can snag your hair out of place. Avoid cornrows, tight ponytails, and anything that pulls your hair back or pins it tightly.

Experiment with loose hairstyles like braids, chignon buns and ponytails to get a fancy look that does not affect the integrity of your locks.

# Treat Frizz Naturally Only

If you have frizzy and untreatable hair, you may think the only option is salon treatments like keratin or straightening. This is the wrong thinking, because these treatments damage your hair from roots to ends and of course causes hair loss.

If you want healthy and manageable hair, change your shampoo. Choose shampoos fortified with protein such as Keratin shampoo to smooth your hair and remove frizz you can use it once or twice a month (every 15 days).

You can also use a protein mask once a month. Instead of using commercial products, create a natural protein mask by mixing two egg yolks in warm water and massaging it onto your hair.

Experiment with protein masks by using bananas, avocados and natural mayonnaise. You can also use leave-in conditioner to maintain shine and get rid of frizz.

# Use a Shower Filter

Taking a shower is commonly known as a cleansing act, but can be surprisingly polluting for your hair. It is interesting to note that you tend to absorb more toxins in one shower than by drinking water. Your skin easily absorbs the water coming from your faucets and shower heads, making shower filters a great idea.

There are many other chemicals such as chlorine in your water that are absorbed by your body during a hot shower as the steam turns them into poisonous gases that are either absorbed by the skin pores or inhaled. An effective shower filter removes these toxins from the water and protects your hair and body.

# Stop Abuse

After you have washed your hair, avoid brushing it when wet and use a wide tooth comb to remove knots. It is best to air dry your hair. However when necessary, use the cool air setting on your blow dryer. To prevent any further damage to your hair, avoid using hair curlers, flat irons or hair rollers that invariably damage your hair.

# Aerating Your Hair

Do not cover your hair too much because you have to let it to aerate, in Muslim countries women cover their hair all time with hijab and that causes hair loss.

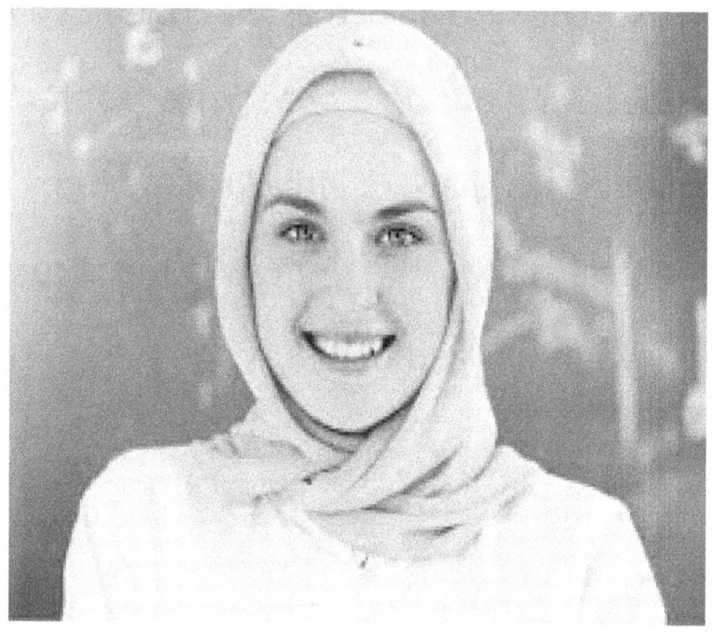

**Hijab**

# a Simple 10-Minutes Regime

Granted you don't have all the time in the world to take care of your hair. But all you really need is ten minutes every day and you can show off lustrous, strong and resilient hair. These simple 10 minutes regime has worked wonders for thousands of women.

Start with a simple health choice by mixing brewer's yeast in the molasses on an empty stomach and drink the smooth. For breakfast, eat a large serving of fresh green salad dressed with lemon juice and proteins for a fulfilling and nutritious start of the day.

When shampooing, use a clarifying shampoo once a month and get rid of impurities in your scalp. On other days, use a natural or homemade shampoo not more than three times a week. Mix your favorite conditioner with a herbal hair rinse as discussed above.

If you are in a hurry and must blow dry your hair, choose low heat settings and place the hair dryer about 5-6 inches away from your head.

Engage in exercise at least 4-5 times a week for about half hour everyday to enjoy better skin and hair.

Don't forget to take your Hair vitamins, rubbing your fingernails and massage your scalp everyday.

Follow these easy tips everyday and enjoy the results in a few weeks. While it may seem a little difficult to fit a hair care routine into your already busy morning, a few extra minutes can work wonders on the health and appearance of your hair.

# Conclusion

At last, you have now all the information you need from diet to treatment options. That will help you to grow your hair and improve your health. All you have to do now is to implement those words and start treating your hair and i promise you will feel massive change. I hope you like the book, stay in touch and i hope all the best for you.


Good luck,


Engy Khalil

# Keep in Touch

**To Read all My Articles and Find the Best Hair Products Please Visit These Websites:**

- Fasterhair.net
- Faster-hair.com
- Hairgrowsecret.com

**Also, if you have any question about your hair or have any question about the program, please contact me here:**

Hairgrowsecret.com/contact/

# Recommendation

## Check out the book preventing hair breakage to get longer hair for best results.

**Please Visit:** <u>Hairgrowsecret.com</u> to download this eBook.

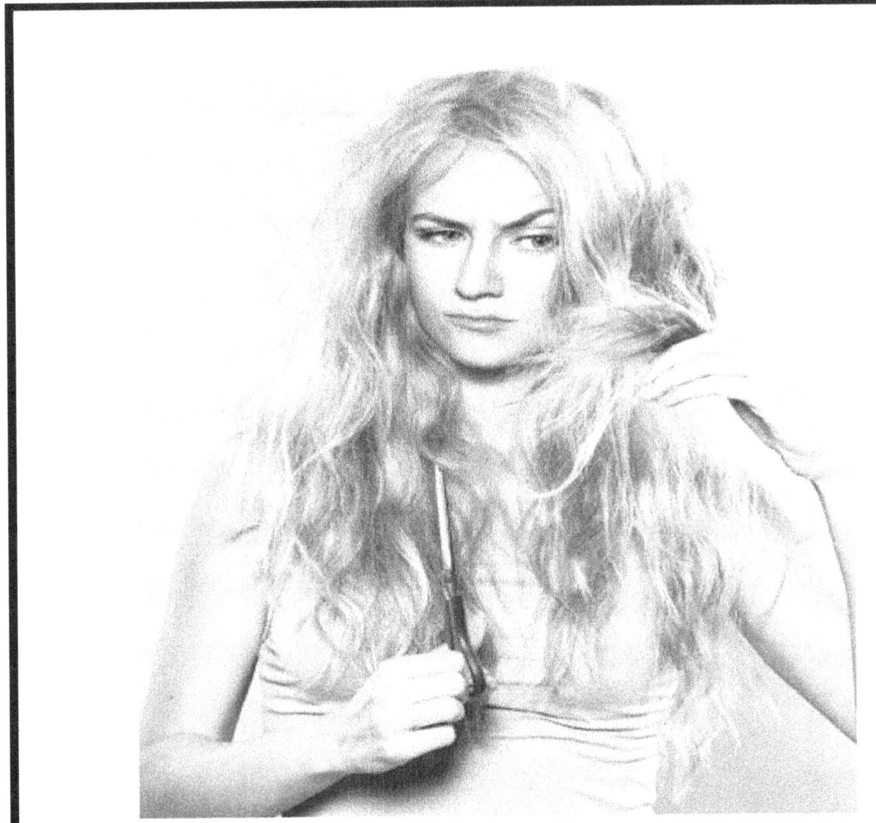